7 DEADLY
INGREDIENTS

The 7's Health Series:

7 Deadly Ingredients: The Hidden Dangers in Your Food and How to Avoid Them

By

Kutu Maurus, M. S

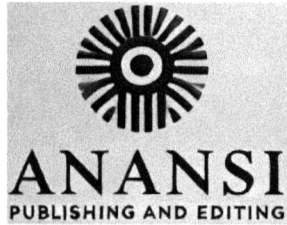

ANANSI
PUBLISHING AND EDITING

2024 ANANSI PUBLISHING AND EDITING

ISBN: 979-8-218-98380-2

Medical Disclaimer

The information provided in this book is for educational and informational purposes only and is not intended as medical advice. The author, Kutu Maurus, is a certified nutritionist and personal trainer with expertise in human nutrition, functional medicine, and holistic health practices. However, this book is not a substitute for professional medical advice, diagnosis, or treatment.

Always seek the advice of your physician or other qualified health providers with any questions you may have regarding a medical condition. Never disregard professional medical advice or delay in seeking it because of something you have read in this book.

The author and publisher of this book do not endorse or recommend any specific tests, products, procedures, opinions, or other information that may be mentioned in this book. Reliance on any information provided in this book is solely at your own risk.

If you think you may have a medical emergency, call your doctor, go to the emergency department, or call 911 immediately. The author and publisher disclaim any liability arising directly or indirectly from the use of this book. Any actions taken based on the information provided in this book are at the reader's own discretion and risk.

"Tell me what you eat, and I will tell you what you are."- attributed to Jean Anthelme Brillat-Savarin

For Nikki, I'm sorry

PREFACE

Nikki was my sweetheart. Nikki was the one I was trying to protect, to look after, to guide. She knew all my secrets, and I knew most of hers (she was much slicker than I was, so she could hide more). Nikki idolized and loved me; I did not appreciate that or know the depths. I had love for her as well, but there were moments when I found myself disappointed with her. You see, Nikki had a struggle. A struggle with food. She regularly hovered around 300lbs on a 5'5 frame. This was death waiting to happen. I was athletic, lean, toned, and muscular. I was, or so I thought, knowledgeable about health and fitness.

I tried to help Nikki by advising her about food and fitness. Nikki's weight struggles created psychological challenges that neither she nor I could figure out. Nikki spiraled into depression, low self-esteem, and low self-love and sadly sought attention in the wrong places with the wrong people. Her low opinion of herself caused her to accept mistreatment from friends and family alike as well as seek continual comfort in food. She continued to gain weight, continued to abuse herself and accept abuse from people. Nikki was the most intelligent of all of us and in another reality, could have been a genius in math or some profession related to high-level mathematics or technology (engineer, etc.).

I got one of those 3 AM calls that all of us dread. As soon as I heard my phone ringing and saw that it was my older sister, I said, "Oh boy, what the hell is going on?". My sister told me that our mother said Nikki was not breathing. I instantly woke, got dressed, and headed down the Garden State Parkway (in NJ) to see about my darling Nikki. While driving, I got several calls, one from my closest cousin, and another from my father. My father was not good at concealing things, and I could tell something was amiss when I said, "Something is wrong with Nikki, I am going down there to see if she is OK". My father made some sort of response that gave me the eerie feeling that she was not OK. My cousin's call sort of confirmed things. She was in an uncontrollable state, wailing my sister's name. I knew what had happened, but continued driving in complete denial.

When I arrived at Nikki's, I saw a lone police vehicle and a county coroner van out front. When I got to the doorway, my niece was crying. I went upstairs, went in, and saw my mother. The officer and another official-looking person were standing in front of Nikki's room door. I tried to bombard my way in, saying, "I want to see my little sister". They denied me this. The next thing I saw, they were carrying her out, wrapped completely in white. "Damn" my sister, it seemed as if all the energy in my body released, and I nearly just collapsed to the floor. I followed them out and saw them shove my sister's body into the coroner's van. They drove off. I uncontrollably ran nonstop until I almost collapsed. I began crying uncontrollably! Nikki, my partner since childhood, was dead, and I FAILED HER. I was her big brother; I was supposed to protect her, and I couldn't even protect her from a candy bar. I had knocked people out for her, protected her in school, and advised her, but the damn candy bars got the best of me, the sodas thwarted me, and the food poisons bested me. When I finally got into Nikki's room, I found a 3-liter bottle of a popular soda brand by her bed. Later, upon autopsy, I learned my darling Nikki had died from a heart attack, all a consequence of her weight. She was 35.

I then vowed to learn the truth about nutrition, food, and fitness. I vowed to help whomever I could live and live well. This book is a part of that vow. There are other Nikki's out there and other big brothers and other loved ones who are trying to help them. This book will help you do that. _Do not do what I did. Do not give up if that person is stubborn or weak and falls short_. The foods are addictive; they are legal drugs, and the corporations and their allies in government know this. They are all accessories. They say you can bring a horse to water, but you can't make them drink". Yes, this is true, but I would add to that and say, "But never stop bringing them to the water because one day they just might drink"

I stopped bringing my sister to the water. My sister visited me that night in my sleep, she said. "Don't be sad, I wanted to die". Well, I am sorry, little sister, but I have been sad ever since. 14 years later, I am still sad, and this book is for you.

Kutu Maurus, Newark NJ July 2024

TABLE OF CONTENTS

INTRODUCTION

Quietly lurking in the shadows of 'healthy' foods, a sinister secret awaits. The media and iconic figures peddle lies, convincing us to devour deadly ingredients that swiftly dig our graves. These silent killers, disguised as 'healthy' options, include artificial additives, dyes, trans fats, and fake sugars. Consumed in large quantities, they lead to a myriad of health problems and premature deaths.

In fact, processed and fast food consumption now surpasses cigarette smoking as a leading cause of premature death (Fuhrman, 2018). Companies deceive consumers by labeling these hazardous ingredients as 'nutritious,' despite research linking them to severe allergies, diabetes, asthma, respiratory issues, and even cancer, hypertension, and stroke. The accumulation of chemicals in our bodies can alter our DNA (Can junk food alter your DNA?, 2022), making these foods a mortal enemy, waiting to strike.

The consequences may seem extreme, but the threat is real. It's time to expose the truth and take control of our diets before it's too late.

This book communicates important information and raises awareness about the dangerous food additives that are intentionally added to the food products we buy. The book deals with scientific facts about what you eat and offers safer, more natural, and real alternatives to eating alternative food.

We have a substantial role to play, choosing organic produce and meat from sustainable farms that treat animals humanely and ensuring regulation of our food ecosystem so we can make informed decisions about what we put into our bodies. This book aims to expose seven universal ingredients that threaten our health once consumed. I hope that by honing in on these "seven deadly ingredients," I will better equip you with the knowledge and insight to make wiser food choices.

Each chapter in the book centers on an ingredient, including refined sugars, trans fats, saturated fats, refined carbohydrates like white flour & pasta, high sodium, artificial additives and preservatives, and high fructose corn syrup. I selected these ingredients because they are commonly present in many ultra-processed foods and have associations with a variety of health problems, such as obesity, compromised immunity, diabetes, cardiovascular diseases - possibly even some forms of cancer.

A choice to divest from these 7 ingredients is an act of self-love and stewardship over your health. I believe that by learning about our food, we would learn to control our health and can live more vibrant lives. This book offers more information than just how to avoid these ingredients, but also why we should avoid them and what products (if any) are healthy and can replace the unhealthy alternatives while satisfying our needs for desserts or cravings.

I have written the 7 Deadly Ingredients book in plain, sometimes humorous language, specifically targeting the casual reader on the move, and it will appeal to even those who have no background or understanding of nutritional science. I hope that reading this book will increase your understanding of the hazards these ingredients introduce to your diet and empower you to make better choices. Busy parents, health enthusiasts, or the nutrition-curious can all learn a thing or two about how to best navigate their way through food and its implications for their health.

Let's make decisions that affect our lifestyle by supporting each other, by choosing to live and let this book help you find the door to good, vibrant health, with one ingredient at a time.

Overview of the Ingredients

1. Refined Sugars:

High-fructose corn syrup, table sugar, and most syrups are examples of refined sugars you would find in sodas, breads/pastries, sweets/candy, or processed foods. Researchers have identified that these sugars deliver empty calories with little dietary value and play a role in the origin of obesity, type 2 diabetes, and other related metabolic disorders. Consuming too many refined sugars causes insulin resistance, which can ultimately result in greater fat storage and inflammation. These, my friends, can be a path to diabetes and heart disease. Later, we will discuss some ways in which these sugars are "hidden" on food labels, making them difficult to detect and avoid.

2. Trans Fats:

The process of using high temperature and pressure to convert liquid oils into a solid creates partially hydrogenated fats, which are very unnatural. Researchers have linked trans-fats to an array of health issues, including heart disease, cancer, immune disorders, etc. Trans fats are attributes of fried foods, simple carbohydrates, baked goods, and margarine; they raise the so-called "bad" cholesterol (LDL) while decreasing the "good" cholesterol (HDL) (Willett, 2017). It is believed by researchers that these fats, in combination with lifestyle choices, play a role in the development of heart disease, stroke, and inflammation-based diseases.

3. Saturated Fats:

These typically come from animal products such as fatty red meats, butter, and cheese, or some plant oils like coconut and palm oil. Consuming saturated fats is associated with high cholesterol levels and an elevated risk for cardiovascular disease. While there are some useful saturated fats, an excessive diet high in these fats may adversely affect our hearts.

4. Refined Carbohydrates:

White bread, pastries, and many snacks are the refined carbohydrates that come from white flour. These carbs are devoid of fiber and essential nutrients that cause rapid spikes in the blood sugar levels to be followed by inevitable crashes. Over time, this can cause insulin resistance, obesity, type 2 diabetes and several cardiovascular diseases.

5. High Sodium (Salt):

One of the biggest causes is a regular or high intake of sodium (usually found in processed and pre-packaged foods, canned soups, and eating out) which contributes directly to hypertension. Chronic hypertension is associated with serious health risks, like heart disease and stroke. To maintain a healthy blood pressure (BP), it is important to reduce salt intake.

6. Synthetic Additives And Preservatives:

Synthetic food colorings, flavor enhancers, and preservatives are artificial additives used to maintain the product's freshness, taste, and appearance. Several costly health issues, including allergic responses, neuro-behavioral effects in children, and long-term health risks like cancer, are linked to many of these chemicals. The U.S. has banned 11 known endocrine-disrupting ingredients from cosmetics, yet the European Union has outlawed over 1,300 (Campaign for Safe Cosmetics, 2024).

7. High-Fructose Corn Syrup

Why would corn, as some studies suggest, be so harmful that it leads to high blood sugar levels? High Fructose Corn Syrup is in most sodas, soft drinks, and processed foods. Because of its high fructose content, HFCS is associated with obesity and type 2 diabetes, partly due to increased liver fat production and the development of insulin resistance, which can lead to metabolic syndrome.

By learning about how these ingredients affect your body, you can become a more knowledgeable and healthier individual.

Structure of the Book

Introduction

Welcome to the wild yonder of industrial nutrition. What you stuff your face with could either be a saving grace or a dismal deadly joke. This introduction is not only a formality — it is a reality check. Buckle up and get ready to dive into seven scary and deadly ingredients that you may or may not know about chillin' in your food, with a side of science & sarcasm (and some light humor). Yes, you will understand more about how these sneaky saboteurs can ruin your life.

Ingredient 1: Refined Sugars

Sugar — the siren that sings to our sweet tooth. This chapter is about the sticky story of refined sugars in everything from your morning coffee to those sneaky syrups that turn up in so many sugary snacks. Find out how they turn your bloodstream into a rollercoaster, spiking and crashing it down, leaving you lusting for more. Sugar Be Gone! I will give you tips to avoid the sugar trap and still keep your sweet tooth.

Ingredient 2: Trans Fats

Think of trans fats as the double agents in your diet—they are forever up to no good. These are the secret agents of dietary destruction that hide in fried and processed foods. They increase LDL, lower HDL, and promote heart disease. Now, do not be afraid. I will give you the knowledge in this chapter that allows you to identify and avoid these villains of fat.

Ingredient 3: Saturated Fats

Saturated fats are like a wealthy uncle who indulges you with sweet treats, but ultimately leaves you with a hefty bill for the consequences. They have flavor and lurk in meats, dairy, and certain oils. If you are looking out for how fattening each one is, this chapter lays down the fat facts (hint: these fats, along with their teammate "trans fats," could jam up an artery faster than you can say "Cheeseburger"). I will assist you in achieving the ultimate pleasure and health balance through lifestyle change - learning smart swaps, moderation tips, and so on.

Ingredient 4: Refined Carbohydrates

White bread and pastries may seem like harmless indulgences, but they are the carbohydrate world's sneaky assassins. The chapter talks about how carbs like refined sugars can slip into your diet and spike your blood sugar before leaving you hanging worse than a bad high five. We're filling your tool kit with some of our favorite whole-grain swaps and meals that will fuel you **and** fill you up.

Ingredient 5: High Sodium (Salt)

Salt is the secret attacker hiding in nearly every food you consume. This chapter identifies the salt in your pantry and how it sneakily raises blood pressure, but we will also discover how to spice your food up (and enjoy the flavor of your food again) without serving a heart attack on the side. We've got your back this low-sodium season, from spices to herbs.

Ingredient 6 Artificial Additives and Preservatives

Welcome to the world of "Franken-foods", home to artificial additives and preservatives. These are the everyday monsters that we consume, especially children, but this chapter will fill you in on the vivid food dyes to the chemical concoctions designed to make your food last forever. I will help you find these ingredients on the label and instruct you on how to replace them with something that occurs naturally. Keeping your food clean keeps you lean.

Ingredient 7: High-Fructose Corn Syrup, or HFCS

The Food World's Skywalker of Dysfunction - HFCS is the supreme, deceivingly polite sweet-talking villain that hides in everything from soda to salad dressing. This syrupy saboteur plays havoc with your metabolism and adds inches to your waist. In this chapter, we give you a road map to avoid HFCS and pick natural sweeteners that are kinder on your body.

Conclusion

In our thrilling conclusion, we sum up the rogues' gallery of ingredients and exhort you to become master of your diet. We combine humor and tough love to equip you for your pantry makeover and help you choose healthier foods. This is not just an ending, but the beginning of your happy, healthy lifestyle.

Appendix

Packed with goodies, the appendix is your ultimate resource. From mouth-watering recipes free from the seven deadly ingredients to meal plans that make healthy eating a breeze, it's all here. Plus, a shopping guide to help you navigate the supermarket like a pro, all served with a side of wit to keep you smiling.

Ingredient 1: Refined Sugars: "The Freindemy"

The Rise of Sugar:

Historical Context and How Refined Sugars Became Prevalent

Sugar is the sweet, seductive siren that has wooed humanity for centuries! Picture this: it's the 16th century, and sailors are bringing back exotic treasures from the New World, including that sparkly, sweet substance that makes everyone go, "Ooh, what's this?" Fast forward a few hundred years and sugar isn't just a treat for the rich; it's the life of the party in every kitchen across the globe.

Once a rare luxury, sugar transformed into an everyday staple faster than you can say "cotton candy." Thanks to the Industrial Revolution, enslavement, colonialism, imperialism, and some very enterprising individuals, sugar refineries popped up like daisies, churning out those fine white crystals by the ton. Suddenly, sugar was in everything from your morning coffee to your evening dessert.

But, like any good plot twist, there's a dark side. The sweet allure of sugar hooked us all, leading to an explosion of refined sugars in our diet. By the mid-20th century, processed foods loaded with added sugars became the norm. Cereal for breakfast? Sugar. Ketchup on your fries? Sugar. That "healthy" yogurt? Yep, more sugar. I mentioned in the previous paragraph, "refineries", you may ask, "What in the world is a refinery, and what happens there"? A refinery is an industrial complex where an industrial process is used to remove impurities or unwanted elements from products such as oil, rubber, and sugar. From a financial standpoint, companies refine sugar to maximize profit regardless of the moral, social, or environmental implications. Therefore, nations experienced colonization or invasion. So colonizers and invaders killed and/or enslaved people, seized lands, cleared them, and prepared them for the production of sugar.

As refined sugars became more prevalent, so did their impact on our health. Those once-rare sugar highs became everyday occurrences, sending our blood sugar on a roller coaster ride that left us craving more. It's like inviting a knucklehead to the party—fun at first, but they always overstay their welcome and eventually do something stupid.

So, here we are in the present day, surrounded by sugar's sweet seductions and battling its not-so-sweet consequences. This section of the chapter will continue to take you on a historical journey through sugar's rise to power, revealing how it infiltrated our diets and what we can do to break free from its sugary grasp.

Ready to uncover the sweet and sticky history of sugar? Let's dive in!

As we journey through the sugary timeline, we encounter key players who turned sugar from a rare treat into an omnipresent ingredient. Enter the sugar barons and vicious detestable slave masters of the Caribbean, American, and South American plantations, where the labor of enslaved people produced mountains of the stuff, making sugar more accessible—and more addictive—than ever before. Picture vast fields of sugarcane, the sweat and toil of countless enslaved people, and the relentless march of economic progress turning cane into crystals.

By the 19th century, it was one of the most profitable industries in the world and you didn't have to be a king or poet laureate to get your hands on that sweet stuff. Sugar started being processed and got even cheaper, making it highly available on every table in the world. Not to mention marketing campaigns that sold sugar as an essential new lifestyle product for the modern family. Advertisements promised vim, vigor, and health—who could resist?

The real game-changer came with processed foods. Manufacturers quickly realized that sugar added sweetness and enhanced flavor, texture, and shelf life. Cereals, sodas, snacks—you name it, sugar made it better. Or so we thought. The convenience of processed foods skyrocketed, and with it, our sugar intake. By the mid-20th century, the average person's sugar consumption had soared to unprecedented levels.

However, with our love affair with sugar came the flip side of that — the expansion of our waistlines. The connection between sugar and a host of health problems was finally inarguable. With the increase in obesity, diseases like diabetes or heart conditions spread. The revelation of the shimmering beauty of our sugar-loving diets tempered as we realized the negative consequences.

So, what now? Understanding how we got here is the first step to reclaiming our health. This chapter not only traces the rise of sugar but also equips you with the knowledge to spot hidden sugars in your diet and the strategies to reduce your intake without sacrificing flavor. It's time to turn the tables on sugar and take control of our health.

Are you ready to play the sugar industry and choose healthier alternatives? Well, get your magnifying glass out; we are diving deep into how sugar sneaks its way in through the back door! But first, we have to investigate why you want it so badly.

Now, picture sugar as the movie star villain — think of an exciting bad boy that everyone loves but should know is wrong for them... It initially seduces you with the possibility of a transcendent euphoric experience. The next bite of that donut and the next sip of cola make you forget all your worries - you're back in heaven with sugar as if it were nothing. However, beneath that saccharine surface lies a con artist playing your brain like a piano with its keys being the slender strings of dopamine. Sugar is addictive because it stimulates the brain to release dopamine (the brain's pleasure chemical). Basically, it will engage in a joyous little brain tap dancing show should you choose to indulge. The problem is that the more you ingest, the greater your brain needs to achieve that same gentle hit of euphoria. It is an eternal pattern of self-soothing and longing (Taubes, 2016), (Moss, 2013). Although your taste buds are rejoicing, your gut is more likely to be screaming.

As you surrender to the sugar siren, it is a game up and down of energy that forces you to reach for more. No wonder studies suggest that sugar, known for its highly addictive nature, can be likened to cocaine. Research has shown that sugar can be as addictive as cocaine (Detrano, 2024). As with any addiction, real withdrawal symptoms occur.

If you try to reduce it, then probably you are going to be irritable, angry, tired, and craving just a taste. A mental battle against sugar ensues, and you face off against it, determined to win. Indeed, this is a challenging situation! But do not worry, it is possible to wage an effective battle against sugar and gain the upper hand. As the saying goes, "strategy defeats even the strongest of villains."

Health Impacts: Detailed Discussion on Obesity, Diabetes, and Other Diseases Linked to Sugar

My friends, buckle up! We're about to dive into the murky waters of sugar's dark side, where sweet dreams turn into health nightmares. Meet the "Freindemy" - the sweet friend who's actually an enemy. Let's start with the heavyweight champ of diet-related dilemmas: obesity. Picture this: sugar is like that charming party guest who keeps offering you calorie-laden hors d'oeuvres, whispering, "Just one more." Before you know it, your waistline has expanded, and your jeans are plotting a rebellion. But have you ever wondered, "Why does sugar pack on the pounds so efficiently?" Well, it's all about those sneaky, empty calories. Sugar provides a quick energy boost with zero nutritional benefits, leading to a vicious cycle of overeating and fat storage.

Next up, we have **diabetes**, sugar's not-so-sweet partner in crime. Imagine your pancreas as a diligent office worker, tirelessly pumping out insulin to manage blood sugar levels. Now, introduce sugar overload! Your poor pancreas is now working overtime, drowning in paperwork (or glucose). Eventually, it throws up its hands and says, "Fuck it! I quit." (excuse the language, but this is serious). This leads to insulin resistance and, voila, type 2 diabetes. Your blood sugar levels skyrocket, wreaking havoc on your body and leaving you with a lifetime of health management.

But wait, there's more! Sugar is an all-encompassing poison. Sugar does not simply settle with inflicting obesity & diabetes, it's an overachiever. It has also top cast billing in **heart disease**, leading to hypertension and high cholesterol (Lustig, 2012). Picture sugar like a charming scumbag, grinning ear to ear the entire time he pours heart attacks and strokes into your veins.

Inflammation is another. It is the body's reaction to sugar's havoc (Hyman, 2014). Chronic inflammation is a sort of smoldering internal fire in your body, and it can lead to everything from arthritis to cancer. It is like sugar has invited all its garbage goat friends and they are there 24/7 junkyard partying in your body whilst your poor little immune system toils away, trying futilely to get it back under control.

Hidden Sources: Common Foods and Beverages Where Refined Sugars Are Found

All right - detective hats on everyone! Ready for some sugar detective work, where we unmask the sweet saboteurs hiding in your kitchen? Because those pesky refined sugars are like Special Ops assassins. They hide themselves in foods and beverages where you'd least expect them to be lurking! We'll begin with the usual suspects: **soft drinks and fruit juices**. Those sweet sips are essentially liquid candy (or crack) - a mouthful of sugar that hits your tastebuds and causes massive spikes in blood glucose, leaving you with the energy to keep going while forcing every ounce of insulin produced by the pancreas to shuttle all those sugars into fat cells.

But the plot thickens! It is in the very **breakfast cereals we consider** healthy and wholesome, which again are just another sugar trap. Even those who like to pretend they are "healthy" choices can be sugar bombs in disguise. Easy and quick to consume, but often higher in sugar than candy. **Granola bars** are branded as the easy, healthy choice. People feel they are signing up for a cute little kitty-cat, but then it turns out to be a tiger.

Now we move on to the **condiments** aisle. Sure, ketchup and Barbecue Sauce might seem savory, but they are hiding behind sugar together with your salad dressings. One drop, one drizzle after the other and you end up with a lot of sugar within your meal. It's like sprinkling sugar on your vegetables—scandalous, right?

Our bakery area will not be forgotten. Sure, you can easily identify cakes, muffins, and pastries as sugar bombs, but believe it or not, even many whole-grain & multi-grain breads can hide sugars. They wear a glowing aura of health as camouflage to their sugary center.

The **yogurt** aisles are no exception, with even "low-fat" and Greek versions often being sugar-filled imposters. <u>Most fruit-flavored yogurts have more sugar than some doughnuts.</u> Yup, you read that correctly—you made a damn doughnut (excuse the expression again, but this is serious business)!

That leads us to the always & forever: **snacks and junk food** sugar syrups are also used to sweeten up many other unhealthy snacks you would typically not expect it in (crackers, chips, and even savory snacks). Which means sugar is like a magic ingredient of junk food.

In summary, refined sugars are the ultimate shapeshifters, hiding in plain sight in your favorite foods and beverages. Armed with this knowledge, you can now become a sugar sleuth, reading labels and making informed choices to keep your sugar intake in check. So, let's unmask these sugary saboteurs and take back control of our diets!

Hiding in Plain Sight: Sugar by Another Name

Ah, sugar is the chameleon of the culinary world! Just when you think you've got it cornered, it slips through your fingers under a new alias. Food manufacturers are masters of disguise, and their lobbyists in Washington D.C. often work with the politicians to allow sneaky changes, sneaking sugar into your diet under a variety of names (Moss, 2013; Nestle, 2002) Let's unmask these sugary pseudonyms, shall we?

1. Sucrose:

- The classic table sugar. Derived from sugar cane or sugar beets, it's the white stuff you sprinkle on your cereal. Simple, straightforward, and sneaky.

2. High-Fructose Corn Syrup (HFCS):

- The villain of the sugar world. Made from corn starch, HFCS is sweeter and cheaper than sugar. It's found in sodas, snacks, and processed foods, wreaking havoc on your metabolism.

3. Agave Nectar:

- Marketed as a "natural" sweetener, agave nectar is extremely high in fructose. It's often found in healthy foods but can be just as damaging as HFCS.

4. Maltose:

- Also known as malt sugar, it's found in malted drinks, beer, and some cereals. It's less sweet but still adds to your sugar load.

5. Dextrose:

- A form of glucose derived from corn. Often used in baking and processed foods. It's quick to spike your blood sugar.

6. Fructose:

- Found naturally in fruits, but also added to many processed foods. In excess, it can be just as harmful as table sugar.

7. Glucose:

- The simplest form of sugar, used by your body for energy. Sports drinks and processed foods contain it. It's quick to enter the bloodstream and provide a sugar rush.

8. Lactose:

- The sugar found in milk and dairy products. It's less sweet but can still contribute to your overall sugar intake.

9. Barley Malt:

- Derived from barley, this sweetener is often used in brewing and baking. It's less refined but still adds to your sugar tally.

10. Brown Rice Syrup:

- Made from brown rice, it's often found in "healthy" snacks. Don't be fooled—it's still sugar.

11. Cane Juice:

- Sounds healthy, right? It's just another name for sugar derived from sugar cane. Found in many organic and natural products.

12. Caramel:

- Burned sugar used for coloring and flavoring. It's found in colas, baked goods, and sweets.

13. Corn Syrup:

- A less refined cousin of HFCS, but still sugar. Used to sweeten and thicken processed foods.

14. Evaporated Cane Juice:

- A fancy term for sugar. Found in many "natural" food products.

15. Fruit Juice Concentrate:

- Concentrated fruit juice used as a sweetener. It's still packed with sugar, minus the fiber of the whole fruit.

16. Honey:

- Natural and delicious, but still sugar. Adds sweetness to tea, yogurt, and baked goods.

17. Invert Sugar:

- A mixture of glucose and fructose, found in candies and baked goods. It's sweeter and keeps foods moist.

18. Maltodextrin:

- Starch-derived sugar is a common ingredient in processed foods and sports drinks. It's quickly absorbed, giving a fast energy boost.

19. Maple Syrup:

- Tapped from maple trees, this sweetener is delicious but still sugar. Often used on pancakes and in baking.

20. Molasses:

- A byproduct of sugar refining. It's thicker and less sweet but still adds to your sugar intake. Found in cookies and sauces.

21. Raw Sugar:

- Less refined than white sugar, but still sugar. Often used in baking and beverages.

22. Sorghum Syrup:

- Derived from sorghum grain, it's less common but still adds sweetness to foods.

23. Turbinado Sugar:

- Partially refined sugar with a light molasses flavor. Often found in coffee shops.

24. Coconut Sugar:

- Made from the sap of coconut palms, it's trendy but still a sugar. Often used in baking and cooking.

25. Confectioner's Sugar (Powdered Sugar):

- Finely ground sugar mixed with cornstarch, used in frostings and confections.

Each of these names hides the same sweet truth: it's all sugar, ready to sneak into your diet and disrupt your health. Stay vigilant, my friend, and don't let these sugar aliases fool you! Armed with this knowledge, you'll be a sugar detective, ready to unmask those sweet impostors lurking in your food!

Avoidance Strategies: Tips for Reducing Sugar Intake, Reading Labels, and Healthier Alternatives

Alright, sugar slayers! It's time to build the most powerful arsenal at your disposal for OPERATION: THE GREAT SUGAR FICTION KILL. Think of it as signing your sugar-free Declaration of Independence. Uncover clever deceptions on food labels, make healthy swaps, and wield your knowledge of sugar to empower yourself for the challenge ahead!

Before we dive into the tips and nurturing, it's essential to become a label-reading genius. Nutrition labels are like treasure maps, minus the buried gold. Instead, you're on the hunt for hidden sugars. Be on the lookout for common culprits ending in "ose" (likely sugars) like sucrose, fructose, glucose, sucralose, and high fructose corn syrup, as well as their sneaky relatives: agave and maltodextrin. If the ingredient list reads like a science experiment, chances are you're looking at sugar in disguise.

- **Outwit the Sneaky Sugars**

Processed foods are sugar's favorite hiding spots. Every day, items such as salad dressings and pasta sauces often contain hidden sugars. Go for whole, unprocessed foods whenever possible. Fresh fruits, vegetables, nuts, and whole grains are your best friends. And when you buy packaged goods, choose those with minimal added sugars.

Tip: aim for products with less than 5 grams of sugar <u>per serving.</u>

- **Add a Few Natural Sweeteners**

Swap out refined sugars for natural sweeteners. Honey, maple syrup, and coconut sugar are better choices, but remember, moderation is key. Try using fruit purees like applesauce or mashed bananas in your baking. They add sweetness and moisture without the sugar spike. This moisture and sweetness keep the muffin from becoming too dry while you eat a bunch of that delicious crumb topping (I mean, duh).

- **Sip Smartly**

Some liquid drinks are full of sugar, sodas, energy drinks, and even fruit juices or cocktails are sugar bombs. Choose water, herbal tea, or sparkling water with a slice of lemon or lime. If you need a bit of caffeine, black coffee or unsweetened tea is the way to go.

- **Cook at Home**

Be the chef in your home and make sure you prepare meals yourself! Cooking at home means you are in control of what goes into your food. Flavor with herbs and spices without sugar, for example, cinnamon, nutmeg, and vanilla extract are excellent if you rely on sugar to make your food sweet.

- **Snack Wisely**

Fight the afternoon lull by opting for fiber-filled protein and healthy fats snacks instead. Try apple slices with almond butter, Greek yogurt, some berries, or a handful of nuts. These will keep you full and your blood sugar under control.

- **Gradual Reduction**

Just do not cut sugar out entirely unless you are prepared for the sugar withdrawal symptoms! Wean yourself off sugar bit by bit until your taste buds acclimatize. First, reduce sugary beverages...then snacks and meals.

- **Mind Your Breakfast**

Most of us already know that plenty of breakfast foods are nothing but sugar-laden traps. **Tip**: Try replacing sugary cereals with oatmeal and fresh strawberries or blueberries, along with a handful of your favorite raw nuts in the morning. Blend up a smoothie with leafy greens, berries, and a splash of almond milk for a naturally sweet way to start the day.

- **Practice Mindful Eating**

Focus on your food and eat it slowly. Being mindful when you eat makes you enjoy the taste and texture of your food more, as well as helps determine whether you are hungry, in contrast to eating for emotional reasons. This will help guide you towards more mindful sugar choices.

- **Educate and Empower**

Knowledge is power when used appropriately. Learn about how sugar affects your health and tell this information to your family & friends and post it on social media with a link to this book! Make it easier on yourself by creating an environment to support yourself in not caving into the temptation of eating more sugar when all around you are cake stands and smiles.

Put these recommendations into action to decrease sugar intake in your daily life, steering clear of hidden sugars in your pantry and fridge, and opting for healthier sugar alternatives.

But we are powerful and can fight back against those sneaky sugar "gangstas" and the food cartels that push them! Our mission must be to regain control of our health — one bite at a time.

Case Studies:

Welcome to Case Studies: the place where fact meets fiction, and we reveal what happens behind closed doors when our fictitious friends kick sugar and more! More than just tales spun to amuse, they paint a kaleidoscope of the good and bad sides of what leaving the 7 deadly ingredients behind can get you. We will do case studies of sorts on all 7, beginning now with sugar.

Meet two personalities in this section: Jane, the one scoring a home run in busting cravings; and Bob, who tries but keeps falling short. They will take you on their journeys to help educate and inspire you about how they approach reducing sugar in different circumstances. Brought to you by the researchers in weight manipulation psychology, these case studies portray a narrative of perseverance, illustrating the journey of overcoming challenges in victory and defeat, ultimately focusing on mastering appetite control.

The stories are just fictional, but the lessons behind them are for sure representative of reality. Like they say in movies/cinema, "based on true events", they develop resilience and show endurance, emphasizing the importance of gradual progress - achieving a series of victories over time to compensate for a significant loss - while also interpreting failure mostly as a foundation for learning and future success. Get ready and find amusement in the humorous and emotional moments as we explore the delightful - and sometimes challenging - experiences of our two sugar warriors.

Case Study: Jane's Sweet Escape

Meet Jane, a self-proclaimed sugar aficionado. From morning to night, her diet was a symphony of sweet delights. Breakfast? A sugary cereal that promised energy but delivered a mid-morning crash. Lunch? A seemingly healthy salad drowned in a sweet, sugar-laden dressing. Afternoon snack? A granola bar that had more sugar than oats. And dinner? Oh, let's not forget the dessert—a luscious slice of chocolate cake to end the day on a sweet note.

Jane's love affair with sugar was a roller coaster ride of highs and lows. She felt energetic and happy when indulging, but soon after, the energy dips, mood swings and constant cravings had her trapped in a vicious cycle. Her once-trim waistline began expanding, and frequent visits to the doctor revealed a concerning rise in her blood sugar levels. The wake-up call came when her doctor warned her she was on the fast track to developing type 2 diabetes.

Determined to take control, Jane decided it was time to break up with sugar. But where to start? The task seemed daunting until she met a brilliant (and handsome) nutritionist named Kutu Maurus and discovered the art of label reading from him. Armed with her new knowledge, she ventured into her pantry, where she was shocked to find hidden sugars lurking in nearly every item. To her surprise, she discovered that ketchup, salad dressing, and even her beloved yogurt were filled with the sweet stuff.

Jane swapped out her sugary cereal for a hearty bowl of oatmeal topped with fresh berries. She traded her sugary granola bars for a handful of almonds and an apple. At lunch, she opted for a simple vinaigrette made from olive oil and lemon juice. Her dinners became a celebration of whole foods—grilled chicken, quinoa, and roasted veggies—finished off with a piece of dark chocolate instead of a sugary dessert.

The first few weeks were tough. Jane experienced headaches, fatigue, and irritability—classic symptoms of sugar withdrawal. But she pressed on, driven by the vision of a healthier, happier self. Slowly, the cravings subsided, and she noticed remarkable changes. Her energy levels stabilized, she shed the extra pounds, and her mood improved dramatically. The best news came during her follow-up visit to the doctor: her blood sugar levels had returned to normal.

Jane's transformation didn't go unnoticed. Friends and family marveled at her new vitality, and she became a beacon of inspiration. She shared her journey, encouraging others to read labels, cut back on refined sugars, and embrace whole foods. Jane's story is a testament to the power of making informed dietary choices and the profound impact it can have on health and well-being.

So, the next time you're tempted by that sugary treat, remember Jane's sweet escape. With determination, knowledge, and a bit of humor, you too can break free from sugar's grip and reclaim your health.

Case Study: Bob's Battle with Sugar

Meet Bob, a man on a mission to kick his sugar habit to the curb. Inspired by a health documentary and the promise of a more energetic life, Bob tackled his sugar addiction head-on. Bob filled his pantry with sugary cereals, candy bars, soda, and cookies—the perfect storm of refined sugars.

With determination in his heart and a spring in his step, Bob embarked on his sugar-free journey. He swapped his morning donut for oatmeal, his afternoon soda for sparkling water, and his beloved evening ice cream for... well, he wasn't sure yet. Bob was ready to conquer this challenge, or so he thought.

The first few days were rough. Bob experienced intense cravings, headaches, and mood swings. He stared longingly at the vending machine at work, resisting the call of the candy bars. His coworkers noticed his struggle and offered words of encouragement, but Bob's resolve was waning.

One evening, after a particularly stressful day, Bob caved. He found himself back at the grocery store, loading his cart with all his favorite sugary treats. "Just one more time," "I will start again tomorrow," he told himself. "I deserve it after all this hard work." That night, Bob indulged in a sugary feast, feeling both elated and guilty.

Determined to try again, Bob made another attempt to cut out sugar. This time, he lasted an entire week before a birthday party at the office derailed his progress. The sight of the cake was too much to resist, and before he knew it, Bob was on his second slice.

Bob's repeated attempts to quit sugar ended similarly. Each time he tried, the cravings seemed stronger, and his willpower weaker. Despite his best efforts, Bob found himself in a cycle of short-lived successes and relapses. He felt frustrated and defeated, wondering if he could ever break free from sugar's grip.

Reflecting on his journey, Bob realized that going cold turkey might not be the best approach for him. He sought the help of a nutritionist, who recommended a gradual reduction in sugar intake and strategies to manage cravings. In addition, he suggested seeing someone to help him navigate the difficulties of trying to eat right when surrounded by situations and people doing the opposite. Though the road was longer and less glamorous, Bob found this approach more sustainable.

He learned that failure is part of the process, and that each setback brought him closer to understanding his relationship with food.

Bob's story, though not a shining success, is a reminder that the journey to better health is rarely straightforward. It's filled with trials, and sometimes, a lot of cake. But with persistence, support, and a bit of grace, one can approach even the most challenging battles in new ways.

Bob's case study shows that individuals may encounter challenges in reducing sugar intake, but with resilience and a willingness to adapt, they can still make progress.

On the road to giving up sugar ... or attempting to give it up anyway, not only do we have our internal battles of willpower being flexed — but sometimes those around us can be that curveball spiritually thrown. Get ready for a shocking story about how the people closest to you - family, friends, and loved ones - can sometimes intentionally or unintentionally undermine your efforts to live a sugar-free life.

Meet our hero, who embarks on a noble quest to eliminate sugar from their diet, only to discover that their closest allies - the friends standing by their side - may be the greatest obstacles to overcome. Who can resist grandma's homemade cookies or a well-meaning friend's urging to indulge in "just one little piece"? Yet, as we navigate our lives while pursuing a healthy diet, we often encounter unexpected obstacles. This story sheds light on the challenges of balancing cravings, moral dilemmas, and love lives with healthy lifestyles. It's a lesson in how the quest for health can become a family affair, where collective goals sometimes outweigh individual desires. So, let's dive in and follow our hero as she battles the sweet saboteurs in her life!

We all love grandma's homemade cookies and that well-meaning friend who always encourages us to eat "just one little piece"

Case Study: Sweet Saboteurs
Tawana's Sugar-Free Saga

Tawana embarked on her sugar-free journey with the gusto of a knight on a noble quest. She had her grocery list of healthy foods, a stack of new recipes, and a steely resolve to reclaim her health. The first few days were tough, but Tawana was tougher. She swapped out sugary cereals for oatmeal topped with fresh fruit and traded her soda for sparkling water with a splash of lime. She was on a roll.

Then came Sunday dinner at Grandma's. The family gathered around the table, filled with delicious home-cooked food. Tawana's heart sank as she saw the centerpiece: Grandma's famous cookies, golden brown and oozing with chocolate. "Just one, dear," Grandma coaxed, with a twinkle in her eye. Tawana's resolve wavered but held. "No thanks, Grandma. I'm trying to cut back on sugar," she says, her voice firmer than she felt.

Next came the office birthday party. Tawana watched as her coworkers indulged in a decadent chocolate cake, each bite dripping with temptation. "Come on, Tawana, one little piece won't hurt," her friend insists, pushing a slice toward her. Tawana sighed, feeling the weight of peer pressure. "I appreciate it, but I'm sticking to my plan," she replies, feeling like the party pooper.

But the real test came from her boyfriend, who showed up with a surprise dessert one evening. "I know you've been working hard, so I got your favorite—cheesecake!" he announced proudly. Tawana's eyes widened in disbelief and rage as she began a profanity-laced tirade at him. "M. F, you know I'm trying to quit sugar, you just tryin' to get me to look like yo fat a**!" she exclaims. He looked crestfallen and hurt; his gesture of love turned into a dietary dilemma.

Despite her best efforts, Tawana slipped. The constant pressure and well-meaning but misguided encouragement from loved ones made it difficult to stay on track. Each time she caved, she felt a mix of guilt and frustration. It wasn't just about the sugar—it was about navigating the social dynamics and emotional connections tied to food.

Realizing she needed a new strategy, Tawana had honest conversations with her family and friends. She explained her reasons for cutting out sugar and asked for their support. Slowly, things changed. Grandma started experimenting with sugar-free recipes, her coworkers brought healthier snacks to the office, and her boyfriend found new ways to show his love that didn't involve dessert.

Tawana's journey wasn't perfect, but it was progress. She learned that cutting out sugar wasn't just a personal challenge—it was a collective effort involving everyone around her. Through persistence, communication, and a bit of humor, Tawana turned her sweet saboteurs into supportive allies.

In the end, Tawana's story is a testament to the power of community and the importance of clear communication. She faced her sugary temptations head-on and emerged stronger, healthier, and more connected to her loved ones than ever before.

Ingredient 2: Trans Fats: The "Frankenfood Fat"

What Are Trans Fats?

Chemical Structure and Why They Are Used in Food Processing

Gather 'round, my friends, and prepare for a journey into the shadowy realm of food science. Trans fats, the culinary world's Dr. Jekyll and Mr. Hyde are a sneaky and mysterious bunch. But what exactly are these notorious fats? Let's dissect them.

Trans fats are the Frankenstein's monster of the fat family, created by the ingenious yet twisted minds of food scientists. From a chemical perspective, food scientists create trans fats by positioning hydrogen atoms on opposite sides of the double bond, giving them a trans configuration. This subtle molecular twist grants them their insidious powers.

Picture a molecule performing a quirky dance, its arms outstretched in mischief - that's trans-fat in action. With their unique molecular makeup, trans fats are the ultimate culinary chameleons, capable of manipulating food textures and shelf lives with ease. But beware, for their powers come with a dark side.

Now, you might wonder, why on earth would anyone create these molecular misfits? Well, it's all about crafting food that outlasts your average sitcom rerun. Trans fats are valuable to the food industry because they prolong the shelf life and enhance product stability. They're the secret ingredient that keeps your favorite snacks from becoming a soggy, oily mess. Think of them as the cooler, more durable cousin of preservatives.

Trans fats come to life through a process called *hydrogenation*. Imagine this: you take liquid vegetable oil, add a bunch of hydrogen atoms, and voilà! You've created a semi-solid fat that can withstand the apocalypse. This process makes trans fats perfect for frying foods to golden perfection and giving baked goods an irresistible flakiness. From crispy fries to flaky pastries, trans fats are the unsung villains behind those delicious textures we love.

But, as with all good things, there's a catch. These molecular pranksters are bad news for your health. They raise your bad cholesterol (LDL) and lower the good kind (HDL), setting the stage for heart disease and other health nightmares (Erasmus, 1993). It's like inviting a charming rascal into your house, only to have them rearrange your furniture in the worst possible way.

In summary, trans fats are the product of scientific wizardry (or banditry), created to make our foods last longer and taste better. However, beware! These deliciously deceptive fats come at a hefty price for your heart health. So, the next time you bite into that perfectly crispy snack, remember the molecular mischief that makes it possible and consider whether it's worth the risk.

Health Risks: Heart Disease, Inflammation, and Other Health Issues Linked to Trans Fats

Brace yourselves, my people! We're about to venture into the dark, artery-clogging world of trans fats. These nefarious fats are like the double agents of the food world, promising deliciousness but delivering a sinister payload of health risks. Let's unpack the havoc they wreak on our bodies with a side of humor to ease the pain.

Heart Disease: The Heartbreaker

- Trans fats are the heartbreakers of the dietary world. They sneak into your diet, charming your taste buds while plotting against your heart. Imagine this: they raise your bad cholesterol (LDL) levels faster than a rocket launch, while simultaneously sinking your good cholesterol (HDL) like a lead balloon. This double whammy clogs up your arteries, turning them into a traffic jam of plaque and setting the stage for heart disease. The method by which this occurs is too biochemically involved for a book of this purpose. It's like inviting a charming swindler to a party, only to have them steal the silverware and leave your heart in tatters.

Inflammation: The Silent Arsonist

- Trans fats are also the silent arsonists of your body, sparking inflammation wherever they go. Imagine your immune system as a vigilant firefighter, ready to douse any flames. But when trans fats are involved, it's like tossing gasoline on the fire. Your body goes into overdrive, producing inflammation that can lead to chronic conditions like arthritis and diabetes. It's a slow burn that leaves your joints aching and your pancreas crying for help.

Weight Gain: The Sneaky Saboteur

- Let's not forget how trans fats love to expand your waistline. These fats are calorie dense and sneak into your diet disguised as your favorite treats. They are so sinister to your body; they appear to be natural fats, so your cells accept them as such (Pollan, 2008). They mess with your metabolism, making it easier to pack on the pounds. It's like having a sneaky saboteur who adds inches to your waistline while you're busy enjoying your fries.

Diabetes: The Unwanted Guest

- Trans fats also play a role in the development of type 2 diabetes. They interfere with insulin sensitivity, making it harder for your body to regulate blood sugar levels (Erasmus, 1993). It's like having an unwanted guest who overstays their welcome and disrupts your whole routine. Your blood sugar levels spike, and you're left dealing with the fallout.

Other Health Issues: The Domino Effect

- The damage doesn't stop there. Trans fats contribute to a domino effect of health issues, from liver dysfunction to impaired brain function. It's as if they have a grudge against every part of your body. Your liver struggles to process these artificial fats, while your brain feels the impact of decreased cognitive function (Hyman, 2014). It's a full-scale assault on your health, orchestrated by the molecular mischief-makers.

In conclusion, trans fats are the dietary villains we love to hate. They charm us with crispy, flaky goodness, but leave a trail of destruction in their wake. From heart disease to inflammation, weight gain to diabetes, these fats are the ultimate double-crossers. So, let's give them the boot and opt for healthier alternatives that treat our bodies with the respect they deserve. Stay vigilant, my friend, and remember, not all that glitters is gold, especially when it comes to trans fats!

How to Avoid: Identifying Trans Fats on Labels and Healthier Cooking Methods

Alright, food detectives, it's time to tackle the slippery world of trans fats. These sneaky fats love to hide in plain sight, but with the right know-how, you can spot them and steer clear. Let's dive into the tricks of the trade for identifying trans fats on labels and mastering healthier cooking methods.

1. Label Reading 101: The Trans Fat Takedown

- Trans fats are like the undercover agents of the food world, slipping into your diet under the guise of everyday items. To catch these culprits, start by becoming a label-reading guru. The key phrase to watch for is **"partially hydrogenated 'such and such' oils."** If you see this on the ingredient list, drop that product like a hot potato. Even if the label says, "0 grams trans-fat," don't be fooled. *Products can **legally** contain up to 0.5 grams of trans fat per serving and still claim zero!* It's like finding out your superhero has a secret weakness. Always double-check the ingredients list!

2. Beware of the Usual Suspects

- Trans fats love to hang out in processed foods. Think of baked goods, fried foods, margarine, and even some microwave popcorn. If it's crispy, flaky, or has a suspiciously long shelf life, chances are it might harbor trans fats. Keep your eyes peeled and your snacks wholesome.

3. Healthier Cooking Methods: The Trans Fat-Free Revolution

- Now that you've got the labeling lingo down, let's talk about cooking. Say goodbye to the deep fryer and hello to healthier methods that still deliver delicious results. For frying, swap out partially hydrogenated oils for healthier options like olive, avocado, or coconut oil. These oils not only avoid trans fats but also bring their unique health benefits to the table.

4. Embrace Baking with a Twist

- Love baking? You don't have to give up your favorite treats. Replace margarine and shortening with butter, coconut oil, or applesauce. Butter in moderation is a better option than trans-fat-laden alternatives. And applesauce? It keeps your baked goods moist and adds a hint of natural sweetness. It's like a win-win for your taste buds and your heart.

5. Grill and Broil Like a Pro

- Grilling and broiling are fantastic ways to cook meats and veggies without adding extra fats. These methods allow the natural flavors to shine while keeping your meals lean and mean. Plus, who doesn't love that smoky, char-grilled taste? (However, be wary of some carcinogens in the smoke).

6. Steaming and Poaching: The Gentle Giants

- For a light and healthy approach, steaming and poaching are your go-to methods. Steaming locks in nutrients and flavor with no oils, while poaching keeps proteins tender and juicy. It's like giving your food a gentle, flavorful hug.

7. Roasting: The Flavor Booster

- Roasting is another excellent method to avoid trans fats. Toss your veggies or lean meats in a bit of olive oil, sprinkle with herbs, and let the oven work its magic. You get caramelized, crispy goodness without the unhealthy fats. It's like turning your kitchen into a gourmet restaurant.

8. Stir-Frying: Quick and Healthy

- Stir-frying with a bit of sesame or olive oil is a quick, nutritious way to prepare meals. Use a variety of colorful veggies and lean proteins for a dish that's as vibrant as it is healthy. And remember, high heat for a short time keeps the nutrients intact and the flavors popping.

By mastering these label-reading tips and healthier cooking methods, you'll be well-equipped to keep trans fats at bay and enjoy delicious, nutritious meals. So, grab your apron and detective hat—let's outsmart those trans fats together!

With these tools in your arsenal, you're ready to conquer the kitchen and keep those trans fats at bay. Happy cooking, and may your meals be as healthy as they are delicious!

Common Foods: Fast Foods, Baked Goods, and Other Sources of Trans Fats

Buckle up! We're about to embark on a culinary quest to uncover the sneaky hiding spots of trans fats. These dietary double agents are masters of disguise, lurking in some of our favorite comfort foods. Let's shine a spotlight on the usual suspects.

1. Fast Foods: The Quick Fix Culprits

• Ah, fast food—the epitome of convenience and flavor. Remember, though, it's also a trans-fat minefield. Fast-food places are usually the ones that use partially hydrogenated oils that give the fries the golden, crisp texture, which is the most sought-after.   Burgers with buttery buns and also some breakfast sandwiches can be trans-fat traps. It's deceptive.

2. Baked Goods: The Sweet Saboteurs

- Your local bakery might be a delightful haven of smells, but it's also ground zero for trans fats. Think flaky pastries, buttery croissants, and melt-in-your-mouth donuts. These baked delights often contain margarine or shortening, loaded with trans fats to keep them tender and tasty. Even that innocent-looking pie crust can be a trans-fat haven, turning your dessert into a dietary landmine.

3. Packaged Snacks: The Sneaky Snackers

- Grab a bag of chips, a pack of crackers, or some microwave popcorn, and you might grab a handful of trans fats. These snacks often rely on partially hydrogenated oils to maintain their crunch and shelf life. It's like a stealthy snack attack, where your favorite munchies betray you with every bite.

4. Margarine and Shortening: The Cooking Conspirators

- Once people hailed margarine and shortening as healthier alternatives to butter, but they often contain high levels of trans fats. They're used in baking, frying, and spreading, making them key players in the trans-fat conspiracy. Whether you're whipping up cookies or frying an egg, these fats can sneak into your recipes and onto your plate.

5. Frozen Pizzas: The Convenience Culprits

- Frozen pizzas are a quick dinner fix, but they often come with a side of trans fats. From the crispy crust to the savory toppings, partially hydrogenated oils are used to keep everything tasty and freezer-friendly. It's like inviting a convenient culinary culprit into your home.

6. Non-Dairy Creamers: The Coffee Conundrum

- That creamy addition to your morning coffee might be more sinister than you think. Non-dairy creamers often contain trans fats to give them that rich texture. Your morning cup of joe becomes a sneaky source of unhealthy fats, starting your day off on the wrong foot.

7. Ready-to-Use Doughs: The Timesaving Traps

- Premade doughs for cookies, biscuits, and pie crusts are time-savers, but they're also trans-fat troves. These doughs often use partially hydrogenated oils to maintain their consistency and flavor, turning your homemade efforts into a trans-fat filthy feast.

8. Candy and Confectionery: The Sweet Saboteurs

- Some candies and confectionery items use trans fats to maintain their texture and prolong shelf life. That chewy caramel or creamy fudge might be more than just a sweet treat —it could be a sneaky source of trans fats.

9. Instant Noodles: The Quick Meal Miscreants

- Instant noodles are a staple for quick meals, but they often contain trans fats in the seasoning packets or the fried noodles themselves. It's a quick meal that delivers a hefty dose of unhealthy fats along with convenience.

By identifying these common culprits, you're one step closer to a trans-fat-free life. Remember, the key to outsmarting these dietary deceivers is vigilance and making healthier choices. So, next time you reach for a quick bite or a sweet treat, think twice and check those labels! Stay sharp, stay informed, and keep those trans fats out of your diet! Happy eating, my friend!

Case Study - Personal Story:
Someone Who Avoided Trans Fats
and the Health Benefits Experienced

Sarah is a 45-year-old marketing executive who came by to tell me she used to live life in the fast lane—and eat in it too. Because what she ate was a fast-food fest; golden donuts and salty fries, buttery pastries - that truly were the best! With her busy lifestyle, convenience was key and her body a domain in empty calories.

It was overwhelming exhaustion, wrapped up like cling wrap, and one day her pants felt tighter than they ever had before the doctor started the 'we need to talk' conversation with Sarah.

The bloodwork returned with extremely high LDL cholesterol (the evil kind) and outrageously low levels of the HDL variety. Her doctor was also brutally honest: "Sarah, you have a diet that is essentially Heart Disease City."

Sarah was on a mission to eliminate trans fats from her diet and set it upon herself to rewrite the health story. With a magnifying glass (basically), she inspected food labels like a noir detective, crossing anything off the list that says, "partially hydrogenated oils." She replaced quick fast-food runs with home-cooked escapades and swapped cherished pastries for fresh fruit and nuts. Her collection of monounsaturated fats—such as olive oil, avocados, and nuts—filled her kitchen.

The first few weeks were hard. Sarah wanted to eat her old snacks constantly, and meal planning seemed complicated as figuring out a Rubik's Cube. Instead, she powered through, fueled by split-second images of low cholesterol and a long life. As you can imagine, her taste buds eventually adjusted, and she developed a passion for whole foods that she didn't know were there.

Three months later, with a trans-fat-free life under her belt, Sarah was back in her doctor's office. The results? Drumroll, please! Her LDL cholesterol was down, and her HDL cholesterol rebounded from the ashes. She lost that excess weight and had more energy than a squirrel with espresso in her system. He was about ready to stand up out of his seat and give her a standing ovation she had done so well with improving that risk of heart disease.

But Sarah didn't stop there. She became a fat-free evangelist, telling her story to friends, family, and anyone who would listen. She even began a blog full of recipes and the advice she learned from making friends with those dietary devils. And finally, science backed her up: studies showed that reducing trans fats intake could improve cholesterol levels, help to maintain optimal body weight, and reduce the chances of heart disease. Sarah, of course — the American Heart Association fully endorsed her "new" lifestyle (American Heart Association, (2017).

Sarah is now a testament to the incredible power of a trans-fat-free diet on your health. She is now making healthy meals; her energy levels are ridiculous, and she has ever since been sharing the word about what eliminating trans fats can do to people.

If you are thinking about evicting trans fats from your home, follow Sarah's lead. The road will be fraught with desires and culinary obstacles, but it is worth the sacrifice to enjoy positive cancer charisma. To a trans-fat-free, healthier you.

Ingredient 3: Saturated Fats: "The Double-Edged Sword"

Understanding Saturated Fats:

Sources and Types of Saturated Fats

Hold on to your hats! We're about to delve into the world of saturated fats—a realm of creamy indulgence and crispy delights. But beware, for these fats are as cunning as a fox and twice as delicious. Let's unravel the mysteries of saturated fats: their origins, how they sneak into our diets, and their impact on our health.

What Are Saturated Fats?

The bad boys of the fat world are saturated fats, their straight-chain molecules, chock full of hydrogen atoms. They are the biker gang of the fat world, hard and unmovable when cool. They are the reason your butter is solid, and why you get that divine sizzle out of a steak.

The Sources of Saturated Fats: The Usual Suspects

Red Meat: Steak, burgers, bacon — a saturated playground! While a juicy burger or crispy bacon may tantalize your taste buds, it also hardens your arteries. **Butter**- The golden spread that makes toast a delicacy. Butter - the quintessential saturated fat that lends richness and flavor to every bite.

Cheese: From creamy Brie to sharp Cheddar, cheese is a saturated fat blowout. It is the life of the party in your fridge, schmoozing with crackers and wine.

Coconut Oil: The fraud of the tropics - Coconut oil. This tropical-sounding health food may also contain saturated fats, possibly comparable to a stick of butter.

Palm Oil: Often found lurking in processed foods and snacks, palm oil is the stealthy saturated fat that keeps your cookies crisp and your margarine spreadable.

Dairy Products: Full-fat milk, cream, and yogurt are dairy delights rich in saturated fats. They add creaminess to your coffee and texture to your desserts.

Types of Saturated Fats: The Motley Crew

- **Lauric Acid**: Found in coconut oil and palm kernel oil, lauric acid is a medium-chain fatty acid that's absorbed quickly but still packs a saturated punch.

- **Myristic Acid**: Present in butter, cheese, and dairy products, myristic acid is known for raising cholesterol levels—both the good (HDL) and the bad (LDL).

- **Palmitic Acid**: One of the most common saturated fats, found in meat, dairy, and palm oil. It's the main offender in raising LDL cholesterol levels (French, Sundram, & Clandinin, 2002).

- **Stearic Acid**: Found in beef and cocoa butter, stearic acid is unique because it doesn't seem to raise LDL cholesterol. It's the oddball of the saturated fat gang, with a relatively neutral effect on heart health.

Saturated Fats: The Double-Edged Sword

- While saturated fats add flavor and texture to foods, they come with a health warning. When you consume too many saturated fats, it leads to increased levels of LDL cholesterol, the type that clogs your arteries and sets the stage for heart disease. However, it is important to note that not all saturated fats are equal, and some can affect your body differently.

So, there you have it—the lowdown on saturated fats, from their sources to their molecular makeup. They're the culinary conundrum that makes food delicious yet dangerous. Enjoy them in moderation, and you'll keep both your taste buds and your heart happy.

Impact on Health: Relationship with Cardiovascular Disease and Cholesterol Levels

Ah, saturated fats—the culinary Casanovas that make our taste buds swoon but our hearts groan. While they add flavor and richness to our favorite dishes, these fats are also the prime suspects in cardiovascular diseases and cholesterol chaos. Let's delve into the tangled love-hate relationship between saturated fats, cholesterol levels, and heart health.

Cholesterol: The Good, the Bad, and the Ugly

- Imagine cholesterol as a bustling highway system in your bloodstream. You've got your good cholesterol (HDL) zipping around like efficient little Ubers, picking up excess cholesterol and delivering it to the liver for disposal. Then there's the bad cholesterol (LDL), the beat-up delivery trucks that drop off cholesterol at your artery walls, causing traffic jams and roadblocks. Saturated fats are the mischievous mechanics who tune up those LDL trucks, making them more efficient at clogging up your arteries.

Heart Disease: The Cardiovascular Conundrum

- Here's where things get serious. Consuming excessive saturated fats can significantly raise your LDL cholesterol levels, increasing the risk of cardiovascular disease. Imagine your arteries as smooth, unobstructed tunnels. As LDL cholesterol builds up, it's like tossing debris into those tunnels, narrowing the passageways and forcing your heart to work overtime. This buildup, known as plaque, can lead to heart attacks, strokes, and other heart-related horrors.

The Double-Edged Sword: Saturated Fats' Role

- But it's not all doom and gloom. The relationship between saturated fats and heart health isn't entirely straightforward. While excessive consumption is an obvious risk factor for cardiovascular disease, the body may need some saturated fats for essential functions. They help with hormone production, cell structure, and nutrient absorption. The key is moderation—finding the sweet spot where you enjoy the flavors of life without tipping the scales towards heart disease.

Scientific Insights: The Evidence Speaks

- Research has shown a strong link between high intake of saturated fats and elevated LDL cholesterol levels. Studies, like those from the American Heart Association, recommend limiting saturated fat intake to reduce the risk of heart disease (American Heart Association, 2021). However, the role of different saturated fats is still a hot topic in nutritional science. (Teicholz, 2014).

Balancing Act: Moderation is Key

- So, how do you navigate this nutritional minefield? By striking a balance. Enjoy your butter, cheese, and steak, but in moderation. Pair them with heart-healthy fats like those found in olive oil, avocados, and nuts. This balanced approach can help keep your cholesterol levels in check and your arteries clear.

In summary, saturated fats are the flavorful foes of heart health, raising LDL cholesterol and paving the way for cardiovascular disease. But with a mindful approach, you can savor the richness they bring to your diet without sacrificing your heart's well-being. So, go ahead, indulge a little—just monitor those LDL trucks and make sure your HDL Ubers are working overtime. Stay heart-smart and enjoy your culinary journey with a dash of humor and a sprinkle of moderation!

Dietary Guidelines: Recommended Intake and the Role of Saturated Fats in a Balanced Diet

- Alright, food aficionados, let's talk about dietary guidelines and discuss how much saturated fats we should eat. These fats can be unhealthy in large amounts. Experts recommend limits on saturated fats. Following these guidelines can help maintain a healthy diet. Saturated fats may be the flavor heroes in your kitchen, but too much of a good thing can turn into a culinary catastrophe. Now, let's explore the recommended intake and how to balance these fats in your diet.

The Golden Rule: Moderation is Key

- Picture your diet as a well-oiled machine. Saturated fats are like the seasoning that brings everything together, but too much, you'll gum up the works. According to the American Heart Association, saturated fats should make up less than 10% of your daily caloric intake (American Heart Association, 2021). For the average adult, that's about 20 grams a day. Think of it as a sprinkle, not a pour.

Balancing Act: The Dietary Juggle

- So, how do you juggle enjoying the rich, buttery goodness while keeping your heart in check? It's all about balance. Your diet should be a harmonious blend of different fats, with saturated fats playing a supporting role, not the lead. Healthy fats like those found in olive oil, avocados, nuts, and fish should take center stage, providing essential nutrients without the cardiovascular drama.

Know Your Fats: The Good, the Bad, and the Delicious

- While saturated fats can raise LDL cholesterol levels, they're not the only fats in town. Unsaturated fats

—both monounsaturated and polyunsaturated—are the heroes that help reduce bad cholesterol and provide heart-protective benefits. Omega-3 fatty acids, found in fatty fish like salmon and flaxseeds, are beneficial.

- It's like casting the perfect ensemble for a blockbuster diet.

The Role of Saturated Fats: Flavor and Function

- Saturated fats aren't all bad—they have their place in a balanced diet. They add flavor, texture, and satiety to foods. Plus, they play a role in hormone production, nutrient absorption, and maintaining cell membranes. The trick is to enjoy them in moderation, savoring the taste without overindulging. Think of them as the spice that enhances your culinary masterpiece, not the main ingredient.

Smart Swaps: Making Healthier Choices

- To keep your saturated fat intake in check, consider making smart swaps. Use another monounsaturated fat oil instead of butter for cooking. Choose lean cuts of meat and opt for low-fat or fat-free dairy products. For more information on healthy oil options, visit the American Heart Association's (AHA) website (2023). Snack on nuts and seeds instead of chips and incorporate more plant-based meals into your diet. It's like upgrading your diet to the deluxe package without losing the flavor.

Cooking Tips: Healthier Methods

- When cooking, opt for methods that require less added fat, like grilling, baking, steaming, or poaching. These techniques allow the natural flavors of your ingredients to shine without drowning them in saturated fats. When you choose to use fats, choose heart-healthy oils like olive or canola oil. Your taste buds and your heart will thank you.

Mindful Eating: Enjoying Every Bite

- Finally, practice mindful eating. Savor each bite, appreciate the flavors, and listen to your body's hunger and fullness cues. This approach helps you enjoy your meals more and prevents overeating. It's about finding joy in your food while maintaining a healthy balance.

In summary, saturated fats have their place in a balanced diet, adding richness and flavor. The key is self-control—keeping your intake below 10% of your daily calories and balancing them with healthier fats. By making smart choices and practicing mindful eating, you can enjoy the best of both worlds: delicious meals and a healthy heart. Stay balanced, stay healthy, and savor the journey, pal!

Alternatives: Healthier Fats to Include in your diet such as unsaturated fats

Alright, let's embark on a culinary quest to find healthier fat alternatives that keep our taste buds dancing and our hearts happy. While saturated fats might be the rock stars of flavor, unsaturated fats are the unsung heroes that make our diets both delicious and nutritious. Let's see these healthy fat champions and discover how to include them in our meals.

1. Olive Oil: The Liquid Gold

- Olive oil is the Beyoncé of healthy fats—versatile, smooth, and adored worldwide. Packed with monounsaturated fats, it helps reduce bad cholesterol and inflammation. Drizzle it over salads, use it for sautéing, or dip your bread in it. It's like a Mediterranean vacation in a bottle! Avoid frying with it, however, when heated, the chemical composition of it changes into something you do not want (Salvador, Aranda, & Fregapane, 2001).

2. Avocados: The Creamy Dream

- Avocados are nature's buttery gift, filled with heart-healthy monounsaturated fats. Spread it on toast, mash it into guacamole, or slice it onto salads. Each bite is a creamy dream that nourishes your body while tantalizing your taste buds.

3. Nuts and Seeds: The Crunchy Crew

- Almonds, walnuts, Brazil nuts, chia seeds, and flaxseeds are all members of the crunchy crew of healthy fats. These little powerhouses are rich in omega-3 and omega-6 fatty acids, which support heart health and brain function. They are not bad in terms of protein either. Sprinkle them on yogurt, add them to smoothies, or enjoy them as a snack. It's like a nutritional treasure hunt in every handful!

4. Fatty Fish: The Omega-3 Warriors

- Salmon, mackerel, sardines, and trout are the omega-3 warriors of the sea. These fish contain polyunsaturated fats that help lower blood pressure and reduce the risk of heart disease. Grill them, bake them, or throw them into a hearty stew. Your heart will do a happy dance with every bite.

5. Canola Oil: The Cooking Companion

- Canola oil is a versatile cooking companion with a high smoke point, making it perfect for frying and baking. Rich in monounsaturated fats and omega-3s, it's a healthier alternative to butter and other saturated fats. Use it for roasting veggies or making stir-fries. It's the secret weapon of health-conscious cooks. Be wary of GMOs in canola, however, stick with the non-GMO verified label if possible.

6. Flaxseed Oil: The Nutty Nutrient

- Flaxseed oil is a nutty, nutrient-rich oil that's high in omega-3 fatty acids. It's great for salad dressings, smoothies, and drizzling overcooked vegetables. Just remember, it's sensitive to heat, so keep it cool to preserve its benefits. It's like liquid sunshine in your diet.

7. Nut Butters: The Smooth Operators

- Peanut butter, almond butter, and cashew butter are smooth operators for healthy fats. Spread them on toast, blend them into smoothies, or dip fruit into them for a tasty, satisfying treat. They're the perfect mix of creamy goodness and nutritional punch.

8. Dark Chocolate: The Sweet Surprise

- Yes, you read that right—dark chocolate can be a source of healthy fats! **Look for chocolate with at least 70% cocoa content**. It's rich in antioxidants and monounsaturated fats. Enjoy a square or two as a sweet, heart-healthy indulgence. It's the guilt-free treat we all need.

9. Tofu and Soy Products: The Plant-Based Proteins

- Tofu and soy-based products are excellent sources of polyunsaturated fats, especially for plant-based eaters. Add tofu to stir-fries, soups, or salads for a protein-packed, heart-healthy boost. It's a versatile, vegetarian-friendly fat alternative.

By incorporating these healthier fats into your diet, you can enjoy delicious meals that support your heart health and overall well-being. So, next time you're in the kitchen, reach for these nutritious alternatives and cook up something wonderful! Embrace these healthy fats, my friend, and let your culinary creativity shine. Happy cooking and eating!

Case Study: A Transformational Story of an Individual Reducing Saturated Fat Intake

Meet Mensa, a 50-year-old professor whose diet was a love letter to all things rich and buttery. Think sizzling bacon for breakfast, creamy cheese-laden sandwiches for lunch, and succulent steaks for dinner. Mensa's motto was "Go big or go home," and his saturated fat intake was off the charts.

One day, Mensa's doctor gave him a wake-up call that felt like a punch to the gut. His cholesterol levels were through the roof, and he was teetering on the edge of a heart attack. "Mensa, if you don't change your ways, you're headed for trouble," his doctor warned. The idea of heart surgery was scarier than a horror movie marathon. So, Mensa decided it was time to make a change.

Determined to turn his health around, Mensa embarked on a mission to cut down his saturated fat intake. He started by swapping his beloved bacon for an oatmeal-based smoothie featuring bananas with fresh berries. Mensa decided to swap the sizzling sound of frying bacon with the gentle buzzing of a blender and incorporate other wholesome, heart-friendly breakfasts. Switching wasn't easy, but Mensa was committed.

For lunch, he traded his cheese-stuffed sandwiches for colorful salads adorned with grilled chicken, avocados, and a drizzle of olive oil. His taste buds protested at first, but soon they enjoyed the vibrant flavors of his new meals. It was like discovering a whole new world of culinary delights.

Dinners became a showcase of lean proteins and plenty of veggies. Instead of slathering everything in butter, Mensa learned to love the natural flavors of foods, enhanced with herbs and spices. He even found joy in cooking, experimenting with new recipes that didn't rely on saturated fats. His kitchen became a laboratory of healthy deliciousness.

The transformation wasn't just in his meals. Mensa noticed he had more energy and felt lighter on his feet. His clothes started fitting better, and he even dropped a few belt notches. But the real victory came at his next doctor's visit. His LDL cholesterol had plummeted, his HDL was up, and his risk of heart disease had significantly decreased. His doctor was thrilled and told him he'd added years to his life.

But Mensa didn't stop there. He became a wellness warrior, sharing his journey with friends and family. His success inspired his wife to join him, and together, they became a power couple of healthy eating. Mensa even started a blog to share his recipes and tips, helping others make similar transformations.

Today, Mensa is a poster child for the benefits of reducing saturated fat intake. He's living proof that minor changes can lead to big results. His story shows that with determination, creativity, and a willingness to try new things, anyone can improve their health and enjoy delicious food along the way.

So, the next time you're tempted by a buttery croissant or a greasy burger, think of Mensa and his remarkable journey. Remember, you have the power to transform your health, one meal at a time! Mensa's story is a testament to the incredible impact that reducing saturated fat intake can have on your life. Let it inspire you to make healthier choices and enjoy the journey to better health!

Ingredient 4: Refined Carbohydrates: The "Sweetest Death"

Definitions and Sources:

What Are Refined Carbs and Where They Are Found?

Alright, carb connoisseurs, let's expose the truth about refined carbohydrates—the food world's sneaky impostors. Refined carbs are like rebellious teenagers, stripped of their natural goodness and packed with fast-burning energy that leads to crashes and cravings.

What Are Refined Carbs?

- During the process of refining carbs, the bran and germ get removed, leaving behind the starchy endosperm. This process strips away the fiber, vitamins, and minerals, turning nutritious whole grains into fast-digesting simple sugars (Pollan, 2008). Think of refined carbs as the junk food equivalent of the carbohydrate world—they give you a quick energy boost but with none of the lasting benefits.

Where Are They Found?

- **White Bread and Pastries: Indulge in the fluffy goodness of white bread, croissants, and pastries, but beware - these baked delights contain refined flour, which makes them a top source of refined carbs.** They may taste delicious, but they're about as nutritious as a fleeting sugar rush.

- **Sugary Cereals**: Those colorful, sweet cereals that turn your milk into a rainbow of flavors? Yep, they're packed with refined carbs. They promise a fun breakfast but deliver a mid-morning energy crash.

- **White Rice**: While rice is a staple in many diets, white rice is the refined version, missing the fiber and nutrients found in brown rice. It's the white knight that lacks the armor of nutrition.

- **Pasta:** Manufacturers usually make spaghetti, macaroni, and all those pasta shapes we love from refined flour. They're quick to cook and even quicker to spike your blood sugar.

- **Snacks and Crackers**: Those convenient snack packs and crispy crackers? Most manufacturers make them from refined grains, making them an easy source of refined carbs. They're the sneaky snacks that keep you reaching for more.

- **Cookies and Cakes**: Desserts are a refined carb paradise. From cookies to cakes to donuts, these sweet treats contain high amounts of refined sugars and flour. They're the siren song of the carb world, calling you in for a sugary fix.

- **Sweetened Beverages**: Sodas, fruit juices, and sweetened teas are liquid refined carbs. They might quench your thirst temporarily, but they leave you wanting more and more. It's like drinking candy.

- **Instant Noodles:** Typically made from refined flours and often come with a side of unhealthy fats and sodium, making them quick and easy, but not the healthiest option. They're convenience food with a hidden agenda.

Why Avoid Them?

- Refined carbs might taste great, but they're not doing your body any favors. They cause rapid spikes and crashes in blood sugar levels, leading to energy slumps, increased hunger, and cravings. Over time, a diet high in refined carbs can contribute to weight gain, type 2 diabetes, and heart disease. It's like inviting a saboteur to your health party.

To sum it up, refined carbs are the stripped-down, fast-burning carbs found in many of our favorite foods. They're quick to satisfy but don't stick around to support your health. Opt for whole grains and fiber-rich alternatives to keep your energy steady and your body happy. Stay savvy and keep those refined carbs at bay while enjoying the wholesome goodness of whole foods!

Health Consequences: Obesity, Insulin Resistance, and Other Metabolic Issues

Alright, brace yourselves, because we're about to delve into the not-so-sweet consequences of indulging in refined carbs. These sneaky carbs may taste like heaven, but they can wreak havoc on your health in ways that are anything but angelic.

Obesity: The Expanding Waistline

- Picture this: you're enjoying your favorite sugary cereal for breakfast, a delicious donut for a mid-morning snack, and a heaping plate of white pasta for dinner. Sounds tasty, right? Well, all those refined carbs are like little gremlins, adding inches to your waistline when you're not looking. Refined carbs cause rapid spikes and crashes in blood sugar, which leads to increased hunger and overeating. It's like trying to fill a bottomless pit— no matter how much you eat, you're never quite satisfied. Over time, this can lead to weight gain and, eventually, obesity. It's the ultimate betrayal of your favorite foods!

Insulin Resistance: The Silent Saboteur

- Now, let's talk about insulin, your body's blood sugar regulator. Normally, insulin helps your cells absorb glucose for energy. But when you feast on refined carbs, your blood sugar levels spike repeatedly, causing your pancreas to pump out more and more insulin. Eventually, your cells ignore the insulin—a condition known as insulin resistance. It's like your body's way of saying, "I've had enough!" Insulin resistance is a major player in the development of type 2 diabetes, turning your love for refined carbs into a risky affair.

Other Metabolic Issues: The Domino Effect

- The fun doesn't stop there. Refined carbs can set off a chain reaction of metabolic issues. High blood sugar levels can lead to increased triglycerides (bad fats) in your bloodstream, raising your risk of heart disease. It's like your bloodstream turns into a traffic jam of unhealthy fats. The constant blood sugar roller coaster can lead to chronic inflammation, which is linked to a host of health problems, from joint pain to digestive issues. It's like your body is constantly on fire, and not in a good way.

Fatty Liver Disease: The Hidden Hazard

- Consuming too many refined carbs can also lead to non-alcoholic fatty liver disease (NAFLD), where fat builds up in your liver. This condition can progress to more serious liver damage and affect your overall health. It's like your liver is turning into a storage unit for unwanted fat, which is never a good thing.

Energy Crashes: The Daily Downer

- Ever notice how you feel tired and sluggish after a meal packed with refined carbs? That's because these carbs cause your blood sugar to spike and then crash, leaving you feeling drained and cranky. It's like a sugar-fueled roller coaster ride that leaves you exhausted at the end.

In summary, indulging in refined carbs might give you a quick energy boost, but it comes with a hefty price tag. From obesity and insulin resistance to a cascade of metabolic issues, these carbs can wreak havoc on your health. So, let's be savvy eaters and opt for whole grains and fiber-rich foods that nourish our bodies and keep those gremlins at bay. Stay informed, stay healthy, and keep those refined carbs in check, my friend!

Healthy Swaps: Replacing Refined Carbs with Whole Grains and Other Nutrient-Dense Foods

Alright, food warriors, it's time to arm yourselves with the ultimate toolkit for conquering refined carbs. Say goodbye to the sneaky vandals and hello to whole grains and nutrient-dense foods that keep you fueled and fabulous. Let's dive into some healthy swaps that will transform your diet and make your taste buds sing.

1. White Bread to Whole Grain Bread: The Classic Switcheroo

- Swap out that fluffy white bread for whole-grain bread (not whole wheat). Whole grains pack fiber, vitamins, and minerals that keep your digestive system happy and your energy levels steady. It's like trading in your jalopy for a top-of-the-line, eco-friendly car—better performance and longer-lasting benefits.

2. Sugary Cereals to Oatmeal: The Breakfast of Champions

- Ditch those colorful, sugary cereals and go for a bowl of hearty oatmeal. Top it with fresh fruit, nuts, and a drizzle of honey for natural sweetness. Oatmeal is like a warm hug in a bowl, giving you sustained energy without the sugar crash.

3. White Rice to Brown Rice or Quinoa: The Grain Upgrade

- Replace white rice with brown rice or quinoa. These whole grains are rich in fiber and protein, keeping you fuller for longer and providing essential nutrients. It's like upgrading from a simple smartphone to a super-smart device with all the bells and whistles.

- **4. Pasta to Whole Wheat or Legume-Based Pasta: The**

Noodle Nirvana.

- Swap traditional pasta for whole wheat or legume-based pasta. These alternatives have more fiber and protein, giving you a nutritional boost. It's like turning your ordinary spaghetti night into a health extravaganza.

5. Crackers to Veggie Sticks or Whole Grain Crackers: The Crunchy Swap

- Instead of reaching for refined crackers, grab some crunchy veggie sticks or whole-grain crackers. Pair them with hummus or guacamole for a satisfying snack. It's like turning a boring snack break into a gourmet experience.

6. Chips to Nuts or Air-Popped Popcorn: The Snacking Revolution

- Trade those greasy chips for a handful of nuts or a bowl of air-popped popcorn. Nuts are full of healthy fats and protein, while popcorn (without all the butter) is a low-calorie, fiber-rich treat. It's like swapping a fast-food burger for a gourmet salad—delicious and nutritious.

7. Cookies to Fresh Fruit or Homemade Energy Bites: The Sweet Treat

- When your sweet tooth calls, answer it with fresh fruit or homemade energy bites made with oats, nuts, and dried fruit. These options are naturally sweet and satisfying without the sugar overload. It's like transforming a candy binge into a delightful fruit festival.

8. Instant Noodles to Zucchini Noodles or Whole Grain Noodles: The Noodle Makeover

- Replace instant noodles with zucchini noodles (zoodles) or whole-grain noodles. Zoodles are low in calories and high in nutrients, while whole-grain noodles offer more fiber and protein. It's like turning your quick fix into a health haven.

9. Sweetened Yogurt to Plain Greek Yogurt with Fruit: The Yogurt Upgrade

- Swap sugary yogurt for plain Greek yogurt topped with fresh fruit and a sprinkle of nuts. Greek yogurt is high in protein and low in sugar, making it a perfect base for a nutritious breakfast or snack. It's like turning your morning routine into a nutritious ritual.

10. Soda to Sparkling Water with a Twist: The Refreshing Swap

- Ditch the soda and opt for sparkling water with a splash of fruit juice or a slice of lemon. It's refreshing, hydrating, and free from added sugars. It's like swapping a sugary cocktail for a sparkling, guilt-free mocktail.

By making these healthy swaps, you can enjoy delicious meals and snacks that nourish your body and keep your energy levels stable. So, go ahead, give your diet a nutritious makeover, and feel the difference! Stay healthy, stay energized, and enjoy these deliciously nutritious swaps!

Meal Plans: Sample Meal Plans That Avoid Refined Carbs

Alright, culinary adventurers, it's time to embark on a week-long journey of delicious and nutritious meals that give refined carbs the boot. Buckle up and get ready for a taste bud adventure that's as healthy as it is delicious. Here are some sample meal plans to keep you fueled and refined carb-free:

Day 1: The Perfect Start

Breakfast: Avocado Toast on Whole Grain Bread

- Smash some ripe avocado on toasted whole-grain bread, and sprinkle with salt, pepper, and a dash of chili flakes. Pair it with a side of fresh fruit. It's like a morning hug from nature.

Lunch: Quinoa Salad with Grilled Chicken

- Toss cooked quinoa with cherry tomatoes, cucumbers, red onions, and feta cheese. Top with grilled chicken and a lemon-olive oil dressing. It would be a lunchtime fiesta in your mouth.

Dinner: Baked Salmon with Sweet Potato and Steamed Broccoli

- Season salmon filets with herbs and bake until flaky. Serve with roasted sweet potato wedges and steamed broccoli. It's like a gourmet dinner at home.

Snack: Greek Yogurt with Berries

- Enjoy a bowl of creamy Greek yogurt topped with fresh berries and a drizzle of honey. It's a sweet treat without guilt.

Day 2: Fuel for the Fire

Breakfast: Berry Smoothie Bowl

- Blend a smoothie with frozen berries, spinach, and almond milk. Pour into a bowl and top with granola, chia seeds, and sliced bananas. It's a vibrant start to your day.

Lunch: Turkey and Veggie Lettuce Wraps

- Fill large lettuce leaves with sliced turkey, shredded carrots, bell peppers, and a sprinkle of sunflower seeds. Drizzle with a light vinaigrette. It's like a low-carb taco party.

Dinner: Stir-fried tofu with Brown Rice

- Stir-fry tofu cubes with mixed veggies in a savory sauce and serve over brown rice. It's an Asian-inspired delight that's easy on the carbs.

Snack: Apple Slices with Almond Butter

- Slice up a crisp apple and dip in creamy almond butter. It's a crunchy, satisfying snack.

Day 3: Midweek Marvels

Breakfast: Oatmeal with Nuts and Seeds

- Cook a hearty bowl of oatmeal and top with chopped nuts, seeds, and a drizzle of maple syrup. It's a warm, comforting way to start the day.

Lunch: Chickpea Salad

- Mix chickpeas with diced tomatoes, cucumbers, red onions, and parsley. Dress with lemon juice and olive oil. It's a refreshing, protein-packed lunch.

Dinner: Spaghetti Squash with Marinara Sauce

- Roast spaghetti squash and top with homemade marinara sauce and a sprinkle of parmesan cheese. It's pasta night, reinvented.

Snack: Carrot and Cucumber Sticks with Hummus

- Enjoy crunchy carrot and cucumber sticks dipped in creamy hummus. It's a snack that keeps on giving.

Day 4: Thriving Thursday

Breakfast: Greek Yogurt Parfait

- Layer Greek yogurt with granola, mixed berries, and a drizzle of honey. It's a perfect way to kick off your morning.

Lunch: Tuna Salad with Mixed Greens

- Mix canned tuna with diced celery, red onion, and a dollop of Greek yogurt. Serve over a bed of mixed greens. It's a lunchtime classic with a healthy twist.

Dinner: Chicken and Veggie Skewers with Quinoa

- Grill chicken and vegetable skewers and serve with a side of quinoa. It's a skewer sensation.

Snack: Handful of Mixed Nuts

- Grab a handful of mixed nuts for a protein-packed snack that keeps you going.

Day 5: Fabulous Friday

Breakfast: Scrambled Eggs with Spinach and Whole Grain Toast

- Scramble eggs with fresh spinach and serve with whole-grain toast. It's a protein-packed start to your day.

Lunch: Lentil Soup

- Enjoy a hearty bowl of lentil soup made with vegetables and spices. It's a bowl of warmth and comfort.

Dinner: Beef and Vegetable Stir-Fry with Cauliflower Rice

- Stir-fry lean beef strips with colorful vegetables and serve over cauliflower rice. It's a low-carb, high-flavor feast.

Snack: Celery Sticks with Peanut Butter

- Spread peanut butter on celery sticks for a crunchy, satisfying snack.

Day 6: Super Saturday

Breakfast: Smoothie with Spinach, Banana, and Almond Milk

- Blend spinach, banana, almond milk, and a scoop of protein powder for a nutrient-packed smoothie. It's green and glorious.

Lunch: Caprese Salad with Chicken

- Layer sliced tomatoes, mozzarella, and basil leaves, then drizzle with balsamic glaze. Add grilled chicken for extra protein. It's an Italian-inspired delight.

Dinner: Baked Cod with Roasted Vegetables

- Bake cod filets with herbs and lemon and serve with a medley of roasted vegetables. It's a fish dish that's as healthy as it is tasty.

Snack: Handful of Fresh Berries

- Enjoy a handful of fresh, juicy berries for a sweet, antioxidant-rich snack.

Day 7: Sunday Funday

Breakfast: Whole Grain Pancakes with Fresh Fruit

- Make pancakes with whole grain flour and top with fresh fruit and a drizzle of pure maple syrup. It's a fun and healthy way to enjoy your morning.

Lunch: Black Bean and Avocado Salad

- Mix black beans, diced avocado, tomatoes, and corn with a lime-cilantro dressing. It's a fiesta in a bowl.

Dinner: Stuffed Bell Peppers with Ground Turkey and Quinoa

- Stuff bell peppers with a mixture of ground turkey, quinoa, and spices, then bake until tender. It's a colorful, flavorful dinner.

Snack: Sliced Pear with Cottage Cheese

- Pair sliced pear with cottage cheese for a refreshing, protein-rich snack.

With these sample meal plans, you can enjoy a week of delicious, refined carb-free meals that nourish your body and keep your taste buds happy. After this week, you will have inevitably gained some ideas and insight for more meals for the week to come. Bon appétit!

Enjoy these meal plans, my friend, and may your journey to better health be filled with flavor and fun!

Case Study: Story of Someone Who Transitioned to Whole Foods and the Benefits They Reaped

Meet Lisa, a 35-year-old graphic designer whose diet was a whirlwind of takeout, microwave meals, and sugary snacks. Her busy lifestyle left little time for cooking, and her health was showing it. Frequent energy crashes, weight gain, and a persistent feeling of sluggishness were becoming her new normal. Lisa knew she needed a change, and after stumbling upon a documentary about whole foods, she decided to give it a shot.

Lisa's first step was to bid farewell to her processed food pantry, replacing it with a vibrant array of wholesome goodness. Out went the instant noodles, sugary cereals, and frozen pizzas, making way for fresh vegetables, fruits, whole grains, and lean proteins. Her kitchen transformed into a colorful cornucopia.

The transition wasn't without its challenges. At first, Lisa felt like she was navigating a culinary minefield. Quinoa? How do you even pronounce that? Kale? Isn't that just a garnish? But she persevered, armed with cookbooks, online recipes, and a newfound determination to reclaim her health.

Breakfasts became vibrant smoothie bowls topped with fresh berries, chia seeds, and a drizzle of honey. Lunches were hearty salads with a rainbow of veggies, quinoa, and a protein punch from grilled chicken or tofu. Dinners turned into culinary adventures with dishes like baked salmon with roasted sweet potatoes and steamed broccoli.

Within weeks, Lisa noticed changes. Her energy levels soared, and the afternoon slumps became a thing of the past. She felt lighter, not just in weight, but in spirit. Her skin cleared up, and she began to glow from the inside out. Even her mood improved —no more angry outbursts or sugar crashes. Lisa was thriving.

But the benefits didn't stop there. Lisa's trips to the doctor yielded impressive results. Her cholesterol levels normalized, and her blood pressure dropped. She even lost those extra pounds that had stubbornly clung on for years. Her doctor expressed amazement and encouraged her to keep up the good work.

Lisa's newfound love for whole foods spread to her friends and family. She hosted dinner parties where she showcased her delicious, healthy creations. Her kitchen became a hub of laughter, learning, and, most importantly, great food. She even started a blog to share her journey and inspire others to make the switch to whole foods.

One of the most unexpected benefits was the joy Lisa found in cooking. What had once been a chore turned into a creative outlet. She experimented with spices, tried new recipes, and embraced the art of meal prep. Cooking became a form of self-care, and her relationship with food transformed from one of convenience to one of nourishment and pleasure.

Today, Lisa is a whole foods champion. She's healthier, happier, and more energetic than ever before. Her story is a testament to the power of whole foods and the incredible benefits they offer. By ditching processed foods and embracing nature's bounty, Lisa reclaimed her health and her zest for life.

So, if you're contemplating a switch to whole foods, take a page from Lisa's book. The journey may have its challenges, but the rewards are well worth it. Your body will thank you, and who knows, you might just discover a new passion for cooking along the way! Embrace the power of whole foods, my friend, and let Lisa's story inspire you to nourish your body and soul with

nature's finest offerings!

Ingredient 5: High Sodium (Salt): The "Covert Killa"

Sodium in the Diet:

How Much is Too Much and Common Sources of High Sodium

Alright, salt enthusiasts, gather 'round! It's time to delve into the world of sodium—the savory saboteur that can turn your diet from delightful to dangerous. Sodium is essential for your body, but too much can quickly become a problem like that overly enthusiastic karaoke singer. Let's break down how much sodium is too much and where those sneaky sodium sources are hiding.

How Much is Too Much?

- The American Heart Association recommends that adults aim for no more than 2,300 milligrams of sodium per day, with an ideal limit of around 1,500 milligrams for most adults, especially those with high blood pressure. To put that in perspective, 2,300 milligrams is about one teaspoon of salt. Sounds manageable, right? But here's the kicker: most of us often consume far more than that without even realizing it. It's like trying to stick to one episode of your favorite show but ending up binge-watching the entire season.

Common Sources of High Sodium: The Usual Suspects

- **Processed Foods**: Oh yes, the convenience of processed foods—ready to eat and often packed with sodium. From canned soups too often consuming far more than that for dinners, these time-savers are often sodium bombs. Check those labels.

- **Restaurant Meals**: Dining out can be a delightful experience, but restaurant meals, especially fast food, are notorious for their high sodium content. That innocent bowl of soup or sandwich can pack more sodium than you need in an entire day. It's like getting a surprise guest at your quiet dinner party—unexpected and overwhelming.

- **Cured and Smoked Meats**: Bacon, ham, sausages, and smoked fish are delicious, but they're also loaded with sodium. These savory treats get their flavor from curing and smoking processes that involve a lot of salt. Enjoy them sparingly, or you'll find yourself in a salty predicament.

- **Cheese**: Cheese lovers, beware! While cheese is a tasty addition to many dishes, it's also a significant source of sodium. Even a small serving can contribute a hefty dose of salt to your diet. It's like a sneaky little sodium ninja hiding in your sandwich.

- **Bread and Rolls**: Surprised? Many types of bread and rolls contain sodium, which helps with preservation and flavor. It's easy to overlook, but those slices of bread can add up quickly, especially if you're a sandwich aficionado.

- **Sauces and Condiments**: Ketchup, soy sauce, salad dressings, and even some mustards can be sodium traps. A little drizzle here, a dollop there, and suddenly your meal is swimming in salt. Watch out for those small additions— they pack a big sodium punch.

- **Snacks**: Chips, pretzels, and other savory snacks are obvious culprits, but even seemingly healthy options like salted nuts can contribute a lot of sodium. It's the classic snack attack—tasty, but treacherous.

- **Instant Noodles:** Yes, they are quick and convenient, but they often contain high levels of sodium, especially in the seasoning packets. They're like a quicksand pit of salt, pulling you in with every bite.

Cutting Back: Strategies for Sodium Control

- **Read Labels**: Become a label detective. Look for low-sodium or no-salt-added options when grocery shopping. Understanding what you're eating is half the battle.

- **Cook at Home**: Home-cooked meals give you control over the ingredients. Use herbs, spices, and other flavorings instead of salt to add taste to your dishes. Your taste buds and your heart will thank you.

- **Choose Fresh Foods**: Fresh fruits, vegetables, and lean proteins are naturally low in sodium. Make these the stars of your meals and snacks.

- **Rinse Canned Foods**: If you use canned beans or vegetables, rinse them under water to remove some of the sodium. It's a simple step that can make a big difference.

- **Watch Portion Sizes**: Even high-sodium foods can fit into a balanced diet if you enjoy them in moderation. Be mindful of portion sizes to keep your sodium intake in check.

In summary, while sodium is an essential part of your diet, too much can lead to health issues like high blood pressure and heart disease. By being mindful of sodium sources and making smart choices, you can enjoy flavorful meals without overloading on salt. Stay savvy, stay healthy, and may you enjoy deliciously balanced meals!

Health Implications: Hypertension, Cardiovascular Disease, and Kidney Problems

Let's go, health detectives, it's time to expose the salty secrets of excessive sodium intake. While a pinch of salt can enhance your culinary creations, too much can lead to a host of health issues that are anything but savory. Let's delve into the health implications of high sodium intake, from hypertension to cardiovascular disease to kidney problems.

Hypertension: The Silent Pressure Cooker

- Imagine your arteries as garden hoses. Now, crank up the water pressure to the max. That's what excessive sodium does to your blood vessels. Sodium causes your body to retain water, increasing the volume of blood flowing through your arteries. The result? Hypertension, also known as high blood pressure. This silent pressure cooker doesn't always show symptoms, but it's steadily wearing down your heart and blood vessels, setting the stage for more serious conditions. It's like having a ticking time bomb in your chest—quiet, but dangerous.

Cardiovascular Disease: The Heart's Dilemma

- High blood pressure is a major risk factor for cardiovascular disease. When your heart has to pump harder to move blood through your body, it strains and weakens. This increased pressure can damage the lining of your arteries, leading to a buildup of plaque—a sticky substance made of fat, cholesterol, and other substances. This condition, known as atherosclerosis, can cause heart attacks and strokes. Imagine trying to drive through rush hour traffic with lanes blocked by debris. That's what your heart and arteries are dealing with. It's a traffic jam that you want to avoid.

Kidney Problems: The Overworked Filters

- Your kidneys are like the body's natural filtration system, working tirelessly to remove waste and extra fluids from your blood. When you consume too much sodium, your kidneys struggle to keep up with the excess, leading to fluid retention and increased blood pressure. Over time, this extra pressure can damage your kidneys, reducing their ability to filter blood effectively. It's like overworking a water filter until it can no longer do its job. Chronic kidney disease, kidney stones, and even kidney failure can result from consistently high sodium intake. It's a heavy burden for these vital organs.

Fluid Retention: The Bloat Factor

- Excessive sodium can also lead to fluid retention, causing swelling in the hands, feet, and legs. This bloating can be uncomfortable and is a sign that your body is holding onto more water than it should. It's like carrying around an extra water balloon inside you—not fun and definitely not healthy.

Increased Risk of Osteoporosis: The Bone Dilemma

- High sodium intake can also affect your bones. Excess sodium can lead to calcium loss through urine, which may weaken bones over time and increase the risk of osteoporosis. Think of your bones as a bank account; you don't want to keep withdrawing calcium without making deposits.

Stomach Cancer: The Hidden Threat

- Some studies suggest that a high-sodium diet may increase the risk of stomach cancer (D'Elia, Rossi, Ippolito, Cappuccio, & Strazzullo, 2012). It's believed that sodium can damage the lining of the stomach, making it more susceptible to cancer-causing agents. It's a stealthy threat that adds another reason to keep your sodium intake in check.

In summary, while sodium is essential for your body, too much can lead to serious health problems. Hypertension, cardiovascular disease, and kidney issues are just the beginning. By keeping your sodium intake within recommended limits, you can help protect your heart, kidneys, and overall health. So, let's be mindful of our salt shakers and make healthier choices for a brighter, salt-balanced future. Stay informed, stay healthy, and keep your sodium intake in check!

Reducing Intake: Strategies for

Lowering Sodium Consumption and Flavoring Food Without Salt

Alright, culinary wizards, it's time to tackle the sodium beast head-on. We all love a bit of savory goodness, but too much salt can turn your diet into a health hazard. But fear not! Here are some savvy strategies to lower your sodium intake while keeping your meals flavorful and exciting. Let's delve into the delicious world of salt-free seasoning.

1. Read Labels: The Sodium Sleuth

- Become a label-reading detective. Scan those nutrition labels for sodium content and aim for products labeled *"low sodium"* or *"no salt added."* If the sodium content looks like a phone number, put it back on the shelf. Knowledge is power, my friend.

2. Cook at Home: The DIY Delight

- When you cook at home, you control the salt shaker. Use fresh ingredients and avoid processed foods that are often packed with hidden sodium. Homemade meals are not only healthier but also more rewarding. Plus, you get to show off your culinary skills!

3. Use Fresh Herbs and Spices: The Flavor Bombs

- Say hello to fresh herbs and spices! Basil, cilantro, parsley, rosemary, thyme, and oregano can add a burst of flavor to any dish. Spices like paprika, cumin, turmeric, and black pepper can also jazz up your meals. It's like giving your taste buds a party without the hangover.

4. Citrus Zest: The Zing Factor

- Citrus fruits like lemons, limes, and oranges can add a zesty kick to your dishes. Use their juice or zest to brighten up salads, marinades, and even soups. It's like a sunshine boost for your food.

5. Vinegars: The Tangy Twisters

- Vinegars are your new best friends. Balsamic, apple cider, red wine, and rice vinegar can add a tangy depth of flavor with no sodium. Drizzle them over roasted veggies, mix them into dressings, or splash them onto grains for an instant flavor upgrade.

6. Garlic and Onions: The Dynamic Duo

- Garlic and onions are the superheroes of flavor. Whether sautéed, roasted, or raw, they can elevate the taste of any dish. Plus, they come with added health benefits. Your taste buds and body both benefit from it.

7. Experiment with Salt-Free Seasoning Blends: The Spice of Life

- There are countless salt-free seasoning blends available that can add amazing flavor to your food. Try blends like Italian seasoning, Mrs. Dash, or create your own mix with your favorite herbs and spices. It's like having a flavor toolkit at your fingertips.

8. Nuts and Seeds: The Crunch Masters

- Adding unsalted nuts and seeds to your meals can provide texture and flavor. Think toasted sesame seeds on stir-fries, crushed almonds on salads, or chia seeds in yogurt. It's the crunch you crave without the salt.

9. Use Low-Sodium Broths and Stocks: The Savory Swaps

- When recipes call for broth or stock, opt for low-sodium versions. They provide the same rich base without the excess salt. You can also make your own broth at home for maximum control over the sodium content.

10. Rinse Canned Foods: The Simple Solution

- If you use canned beans or vegetables, give them a good rinse under water to wash away some of the sodium. It's a quick and easy way to reduce your intake without sacrificing convenience.

11. Be a Smart Snacker: The Savvy Selector

- Choose snacks that are naturally low in sodium, like fresh fruit, vegetables, unsalted nuts, and plain popcorn. Monitor portion sizes and avoid the temptation of salty treats.

12. Gradually Reduce Salt: The Gentle Approach

- If you're used to salty foods, your taste buds might need some time to adjust. Gradually reduce the amount of salt you use in cooking and at the table. Over time, you'll appreciate the natural flavors of food with no added salt.

In summary, lowering your sodium intake doesn't mean sacrificing flavor. With a little creativity and a willingness to experiment, you can enjoy delicious, savory meals without the health risks associated with high sodium consumption. So, grab your herbs, spices, and citrus, and let's make mealtime a flavorful adventure! Stay flavorful, stay healthy, and enjoy the culinary journey!

Recipe Ideas: Low-Sodium Recipes to Try at Home

Yes, food enthusiasts! It's time to get busy in the kitchen and explore some flavorful recipes that are low in sodium but still delicious. These dishes are not only delicious but also heart-healthy. Let's get cooking!

1. Zesty Lemon Herb Chicken

Ingredients:

- 4 boneless, skinless chicken breasts
- 2 lemons (juice and zest)
- 3 cloves garlic, minced
- 2 tablespoons olive oil
- 1 tablespoon fresh rosemary, chopped
- 1 tablespoon fresh thyme, chopped

- Black pepper to taste

Instructions:

1. In a bowl, mix lemon juice, lemon zest, garlic, olive oil, rosemary, thyme, and black pepper.

2. Place chicken breasts in a resealable bag or shallow dish and pour the marinade over them. Marinate in the refrigerator for at least 30 minutes.

3. Preheat the grill to medium-high heat.

4. Grill chicken breasts for 6-7 minutes on each side, or until fully cooked.

5. Serve with a side of steamed vegetables or a fresh salad. It's a zesty, herbaceous delight!

2. Spicy Quinoa and Black Bean Salad

Ingredients:

- 1 cup quinoa, rinsed
- 2 cups low-sodium vegetable broth
- 1 can black beans, rinsed and drained
- 1 cup cherry tomatoes, halved
- 1 red bell pepper, diced
- 1 avocado, diced
- 1/4 cup fresh cilantro, chopped
- 1/4 cup fresh lime juice
- 1 tablespoon cumin
- 1/2 tablespoon chili powder
- Black pepper to taste

Instructions:

1. Cook quinoa in low-sodium vegetable broth according to package instructions. Let it cool.

2. In a large bowl, combine quinoa, black beans, cherry tomatoes, red bell pepper, avocado, and cilantro.

3. In a small bowl, whisk together lime juice, cumin, chili powder, and black pepper.

4. Pour the dressing over the salad and toss to combine.

5. Serve chilled. It's a fiesta in a bowl!

3. Garlic and Herb Roasted Vegetables

Ingredients:

- 2 cups broccoli florets
- 2 cups cauliflower florets
- 2 cups carrot sticks
- 2 tbsp olive oil
- 3 cloves garlic, minced
- 1 tablespoon fresh thyme, chopped
- 1 tablespoon fresh rosemary, chopped
- Black pepper to taste

Instructions:

1. Preheat the oven to 400°F (200°C).

2. In a large bowl, toss the vegetables with olive oil, garlic, thyme, rosemary, and black pepper.

3. Spread the vegetables in a single layer on a baking sheet.

4. Roast for 20-25 minutes, or until the vegetables are tender and slightly caramelized.

5. Serve as a side dish or a main course. It's a roasted revelation!

4. Tangy Citrus and Avocado Salad

Ingredients:

- 2 large oranges, peeled and sliced
- 1 grapefruit, peeled and sliced
- 1 avocado, sliced
- 1/4 cup red onion, thinly sliced
- 2 cups mixed greens
- 1/4 cup fresh mint leaves, chopped
- 1/4 cup fresh lime juice
- 1 tablespoon olive oil
- Black pepper to taste

Instructions:

1. In a large bowl, combine oranges, grapefruit, avocado, red onion, mixed greens, and mint leaves.
2. In a small bowl, whisk together lime juice, olive oil, and black pepper.
3. Drizzle the dressing over the salad and toss gently to combine.
4. Serve immediately. It's a citrusy, creamy delight!

5. Hearty Lentil Soup

Ingredients:

- 1 cup lentils, rinsed
- 1 tablespoon olive oil
- 1 onion, diced
- 2 carrots, diced
- 2 celery stalks, diced
- 3 cloves garlic, minced
- 1 can diced tomatoes (no salt added)
- 4 cups low-sodium vegetable broth

- 1 tablespoon cumin
- 1 tablespoon smoked paprika
- 1 bay leaf
- Black pepper to taste
- Fresh parsley, chopped (for garnish)

Instructions:

1. In a large pot, heat olive oil over medium heat. Add onion, carrots, and celery. Sauté until vegetables are tender.

2. Add garlic and cook for another minute.

3. Stir in diced tomatoes, vegetable broth, lentils, cumin, smoked paprika, bay leaf, and black pepper.

4. Bring to a boil, then reduce heat and simmer for 30-35 minutes, or until lentils are tender.

5. Remove bay leaf and garnish with fresh parsley before serving.

6. Enjoy a bowl of this hearty, comforting soup!

With these low-sodium recipes, you can enjoy flavorful, nutritious meals without the excess salt. Happy cooking, and bon appétit! Embrace the joy of cooking with these delicious, low-sodium recipes!

Case Study-Real-Life Impact: Contrasting Stories of Success and Failure in Reducing Sodium Intake

Meet John and Mike, two friends who shared a love for salty snacks and savory delights. Both were in their mid-50s, they enjoyed bonding over bags of chips, pretzels, and countless fast-food meals. However, when their doctors gave them stern warnings about their skyrocketing blood pressure, their paths diverged dramatically.

John's Success Story

Determined to take control of his health, John decided it was time to bid farewell to his salty ways. He overhauled his kitchen, replacing high-sodium snacks and processed foods with fresh vegetables, lean proteins, and whole grains. He became a label-reading ninja, scouring every product for hidden sodium.

John's meals transformed into vibrant culinary masterpieces. Breakfasts featured Greek yogurt with fresh berries and nuts, lunches showcased colorful salads with balsamic vinegar, and dinners became gourmet events with grilled chicken, quinoa, and steamed broccoli. His palate adjusted to the natural flavors of food, and he no longer craved the intense saltiness of his old diet.

Within weeks, John's health improved. Headaches lessened, energy levels soared, and his follow-up doctor's appointment revealed significantly lower blood pressure. He lost weight, felt more energetic, and even noticed an uplifted mood. John's journey inspired friends and family, turning him into an advocate for low-sodium living.

Mike's Unfortunate Demise

Meanwhile, Mike decided to stick with his salty favorites, dismissing his doctor's warnings as exaggerated. His kitchen remained a haven of processed foods, and his meals were a constant barrage of sodium. Breakfasts of sugary cereals, lunches of canned soups, and dinners of takeout pizza were his daily fare.

Mike's health took a downward spiral. Frequent headaches became migraines, his energy levels plummeted, and his weight ballooned. Ignoring his body's distress signals, Mike continued indulging in high-sodium delights, convinced he could manage the consequences later.

One evening, Mike binged-watched his favorite show with a feast of salty snacks and a couple of pizzas. As he laughed at the antics on the screen, his heart and kidneys silently protested. The next morning, Mike didn't wake up. His heart had given out, overwhelmed by the constant strain of high blood pressure and poor diet. The tragic news of Mike's untimely demise shocked his friends and family.

The Lessons Learned

John's success story and Mike's unfortunate demise serve as powerful reminders of the impact of our dietary choices. John's journey to lower sodium intake transformed his health, bringing energy, vitality, and inspiration to those around him. Mike's refusal to change led to a tragic, preventable end.

While John enjoys a life filled with flavorful, healthy meals and endless energy, Mike's story is a stark warning about the dangers of ignoring dietary advice. The contrast between their lives highlights the importance of making mindful choices and listening to our bodies.

In conclusion, embrace the power of reducing sodium intake. Follow John's lead and transform your diet to enjoy a healthier, happier life. Let Mike's story be a cautionary tale, reminding us that the price of ignoring our health can be far too high.

Stay mindful, stay healthy, and make choices that support your well-being. Remember, these two stories and unlike the old Nike commercials, don't "be like Mike"!

Ingredient 6: Artificial Additives, and Preservatives: The "Lovely Assassins"

What Are They?

Types of Additives and Preservatives Used in Food, Including Synthetic Food Dyes

Alright, food detectives, it's time to uncover the mysterious world of additives and preservatives—the undercover agents in your favorite snacks and meals. These sneaky substances help keep our food fresh, flavorful, and visually appealing, but they come with their own set of quirks. Let's dive into the different types and see what's lurking in our food.

1. Preservatives: The Timekeepers

- **Sodium Benzoate**: This preservative is a staple in acidic foods like sodas, salad dressings, and fruit juices. It's like the bouncer at the club, keeping bacteria and fungi at bay so your food stays fresh.

- **Potassium Sorbate**: Found in cheese, wine, and baked goods, potassium sorbate prevents mold and yeast from crashing the party. It's the invisible force field protecting your snacks.

- **BHA and BHT**: Butylated hydroxyanisole (BHA) and butylated hydroxytoluene (BHT) are antioxidants that keep oils and fats from turning rancid. Think of them as the bodyguards for your chips and cereals, ensuring they stay crispy and fresh.

2. Flavor Enhancers: The Taste Bud Titans

- **Monosodium Glutamate (MSG)**: This infamous flavor

enhancer gives a savory umami punch to soups, processed meats, and snacks. It's like the flavor amplifier that turns up the taste dial to eleven.

- **Disodium Inosinate and Disodium Guanylate**: Often used in tandem with MSG, these enhancers boost the savory flavor in instant noodles, snacks, and canned soups. They're the backup singers, making sure your taste buds are always in harmony.

3. Stabilizers and Thickeners: The Texture Transformers

- **Xanthan Gum**: A polysaccharide used in salad dressings, sauces, and gluten-free products to thicken and stabilize. It's the smooth operator ensuring your favorite dressings don't separate.

- **Carrageenan,** which is derived from seaweed, is present in dairy products and plant-based milks. It's the gelatinous glue that keeps your milkshake creamy and your yogurt luscious.

- **Guar Gum:** This thickener, sourced from guar beans, is used in ice cream, sauces, and baked goods. It's like the magician that transforms liquids into velvety smooth textures.

4. Sweeteners: The Sugar Stand-Ins

- **Aspartame**: A low-calorie sweetener found in diet sodas, sugar-free gum, and light desserts. It's the sweet talker convincing your taste buds they're indulging without the calories.

- **Sucralose:** commercially known as Splenda, finds its use in baked goods, beverages, and chewing gum. It's the sugar imposter that keeps things sweet without the sugar rush.

- **Stevia**: A natural sweetener derived from the leaves of the Stevia plant. It's like the herbal hero offering sweetness with a side of health benefits.

5. Color Additives: The Visual Virtuosos

- **Synthetic Food Dyes**: These colorful characters include Red 40, Yellow 5, and Blue 1. They're the artists making your candies, sodas, and baked goods look irresistibly vibrant. However, they face frequent scrutiny for potential health risks and some countries have banned them.

- **Natural Colorings**: Extracted from plants and minerals, these include beet juice, turmeric, and annatto. They're the organic painters adding a splash of color without the synthetic side effects.

6. Emulsifiers: The Mix Masters

- **Lecithin**: Found in chocolate, margarine, and salad dressings, lecithin helps blend ingredients that rarely mix, like oil and water. It's the peacemaker keeping your food components in perfect harmony.

- **Mono- and Diglycerides**: Used in baked goods and ice cream, these emulsifiers improve texture and shelf life. They're the secret agents working behind the scenes to keep your treats delightful.

7. Antioxidants: The Freshness Protectors

- **Ascorbic Acid (Vitamin C)**: Commonly added to juices, canned fruits, and processed foods to prevent oxidation and preserve color. It's the vitamin superhero keeping your food fresh and vibrant.

- **Tocopherols (Vitamin E)**: Used in oils and cereals, tocopherols prevent fats from going rancid. They're the guardians of freshness, ensuring your food stays delicious.

In summary, additives and preservatives are the unsung heroes (and sometimes villains) of the food world, keeping our meals fresh, flavorful, and visually appealing. While some are essential for food safety and quality, others are best consumed in moderation. Stay informed, and you'll be a savvy eater in no time! Stay curious, stay informed, and keep uncovering the secrets of your food, my friend!

Health Concerns: Potential Risks and Long-Term Effects of Consuming Artificial Ingredients

OK, my beloved food explorers, it's time to venture into the murky waters of artificial ingredients. These sneaky substances might make our food look and taste great, but they come with a host of health concerns that could leave you scratching your head—and your stomach. Let's dive into the potential risks and long-term effects of consuming these culinary chameleons.

1. Synthetic Food Dyes: The Colorful Conundrum

- Synthetic food dyes like Red 40, Yellow 5, and Blue 1 are the life of the party in candies, sodas, and cereals. But behind those vibrant hues lies a world of potential health risks. Studies suggest these dyes may have a link to hyperactivity in children and allergic reactions in sensitive individuals (Schab & Trinh, 2004). Some even raise concerns about carcinogenicity, making these colorful additives less of a rainbow and more of a storm cloud (Blythman, 2015).

2. Artificial Sweeteners: The Sweet Deceivers

- Artificial sweeteners like aspartame, sucralose, and saccharin are the darlings of diet sodas and sugar-free snacks. They promise sweetness without the calories, but at what cost? Some research points to potential issues like headaches, digestive problems, and even an increased risk of metabolic syndrome.

Aspartame, in particular, has faced scrutiny over links to neurological issues (Mercola & Pearsall, 2006). It's like inviting a charming guest to your party only to find they overstayed their welcome and trashed the place.

3. Preservatives: The Longevity Lurkers

- Preservatives such as BHA, BHT, and sodium benzoate keep our foods fresh, but they also raise some red flags. BHA and BHT are antioxidants used in snacks and cereals, yet they've been shown to cause cancer in animals, leading to concerns about their safety in humans (O'Brien & Kranz, 2009). Sodium benzoate, found in sodas and dressings, can form benzene—a known carcinogen—when combined with vitamin C (O'Brien & Kranz, 2009). It's like adding a ticking time bomb to your pantry.

4. Flavor Enhancers: The Taste Tempters

- Monosodium glutamate (MSG) and other flavor enhancers make our taste buds dance, but they can also cause some serious side effects. While the "Chinese Restaurant Syndrome" (headaches, sweating, and flushing) has been largely debunked, some individuals still experience sensitivity to MSG, leading to symptoms such as chest pain and palpitations. It's like turning up the volume to enjoy the music, only to end up with a headache.

5. Emulsifiers and Stabilizers: The Texture Tricksters

- Emulsifiers like lecithin and carrageenan keep your salad dressings creamy and your ice cream smooth, but they might also cause digestive distress. Some studies have linked carrageenan, in particular, to inflammation and gastrointestinal issues (Hari, 2016). It's like having a smooth ride until you hit an unexpected pothole.

6. High-Fructose Corn Syrup: The Sugar Shapeshifter

- High-fructose corn syrup (HFCS) is a cheap alternative to sugar found in sodas, candies, and processed foods. Consuming too much HFCS can lead to obesity, insulin resistance, and type 2 diabetes. It's like swapping your regular fuel for a cheaper, dirtier version that clogs up your engine over time. We will discuss HFCS in the next ingredient chapter.

7. Trans Fats: The Hidden Heartbreakers

- Partially hydrogenated oils, aka trans fats, are used to extend shelf life and improve texture in baked goods and margarine. These fats raise bad cholesterol (LDL) and lower good cholesterol (HDL), increasing the risk of heart disease. It's like inviting a smooth-talking villain into your home, only to find out they've been robbing you blind. We have discussed this previously in this book.

8. Additives and Asthma: The Breathing Baddies

- Certain additives, like sulfites used in wine and dried fruits, can trigger asthma symptoms and allergic reactions (Statham, 2007). It's like enjoying your favorite treats only to find yourself gasping for breath.

In summary, while artificial ingredients make our food more convenient, colorful, and flavorful, they come with a laundry list of potential health risks. From hyperactivity and allergic reactions to more serious concerns like cancer and heart disease, these additives are best consumed with caution. Stay informed, read labels, and opt for natural alternatives whenever possible. Your body will thank you! Stay savvy, stay healthy, and navigate the world of artificial ingredients with a discerning eye, beloved.

Identifying Additives: How to Read Labels and Avoid Harmful Additives

It's time to become the Sherlock Holmes of the grocery store aisles. The world of food labels contains mysterious additives, cryptic codes, and ingredients that sound like they belong in a chemistry lab. Fear not! With a keen eye and a bit of know-how, you can decipher these labels and dodge harmful additives like a pro. Let's dive into the art of identifying additives and making smarter food choices.

1. The Ingredient List: The Additive Encyclopedia

- The first step in your detective work is to scan the ingredient list. Ingredients are listed in descending order by weight, so the first few items are the most abundant. Keep an eye out for long lists filled with unpronounceable words—these are often red flags for additives and preservatives.

2. Beware of the Usual Suspects

- **Artificial Sweeteners**: Look for names like aspartame, sucralose, and saccharin. These sweet talkers can hide in diet sodas, sugar-free gum, and low-calorie snacks.

- **Synthetic Food Dyes**: Keep an eye out for Red 40, Yellow 5 & 6, and Blue 1. These colorful characters are common in candies, sodas, and baked goods.

- **Preservatives**: Sodium benzoate, potassium sorbate, and BHA/BHT are common preservatives found in processed foods, snacks, and beverages.

- **Flavor Enhancers**: Monosodium glutamate (MSG) and disodium inosinate are often found in savory snacks, soups, and processed meats.

3. Decode the Additive Aliases

- Additives often go by multiple names. For example,

MSG may appear on the list as monosodium glutamate, hydrolyzed protein, or autolyzed yeast extract. Familiarize yourself with these aliases to spot them more easily.

4. Look for Natural Alternatives

- Choose products with natural ingredients like cane sugar instead of high-fructose corn syrup, or beet juice for coloring instead of synthetic dyes. If the ingredients sound like something you'd find in your kitchen, you're on the right track.

5. Check for Certifications

- Look for certifications like USDA Organic or Non-GMO Project Verified. These labels show the product meets certain standards for natural ingredients and minimal processing. It's like a stamp of approval from Mother Nature herself.

6. Avoid the Numbers Game

- Additives often come with cryptic numbers, like E320 (BHA) or E621 (MSG). Familiarize yourself with these codes and avoid products that list them. It's like playing a game of bingo where you want to avoid shouting "E-numbers!"

7. Shop the Perimeter

- The healthiest foods, such as fresh fruits, vegetables, meats, and dairy, are typically located around the perimeter of the grocery store. Processed foods and their additive friends hang out in the middle aisles.

8. DIY: The Ultimate Control

- Make your own meals and snacks from scratch. This gives you complete control over what goes into your food. Plus, it's a great way to unleash your inner chef and impress your friends with your culinary prowess.

9. Use Apps and Resources

- Several apps and websites can help you decode food labels and identify harmful additives. Apps like Fooducate and EWG's Food Scores provide detailed information on ingredients and their health effects.

10. Trust Your Gut

- If you come across an ingredient you don't recognize, look it up before buying. Trust your instincts—if it sounds like it belongs in a science experiment, it's probably best to avoid it.

In summary, reading labels and identifying additives is a crucial skill for navigating the modern food landscape. By becoming a savvy label reader and making informed choices, you can avoid harmful additives and enjoy a healthier diet. So, grab your magnifying glass, channel your inner detective, and let's crack the case of the mysterious additives! Stay curious, stay informed, and master the art of label reading, friend!

Natural Alternatives: Using Natural Preservatives and Making Homemade Versions of Common Foods

My kitchen alchemists, it's time to embrace the power of nature and transform your culinary creations with natural preservatives and homemade versions of your favorite foods. Say goodbye to artificial additives and hello to wholesome goodness that's as tasty as it is nourishing. Let's dive into the world of natural alternatives and homemade magic.

1. Lemon Juice: The Zesty Preserver

- Lemon juice is a powerhouse of natural preservation, thanks to its high acidity and vitamin C content. It's perfect for keeping fruits like apples and avocados from turning brown. Just a splash can work wonders in salad dressings, marinades, and even baked goods. It's like adding a zesty superhero to your kitchen arsenal.

2. Vinegar: The Tangy Guardian

- Vinegar, especially apple cider and white vinegar, is a fantastic natural preservative. Its acidity helps prevent spoilage and bacterial growth. Use it in pickling vegetables, making sauces, or as a natural cleaning agent. It's the tangy guardian that keeps your food fresh and your kitchen sparkling.

3. Honey: The Sweet Protector

- Honey isn't just delicious; it's also a natural preservative with antimicrobial properties. It's perfect for sweetening and preserving jams, jellies, and sauces. Plus, it's a great alternative to sugar in baking. It's like nature's golden syrup that keeps your treats sweet and safe.

4. Salt: The Classic Preserver

- Ancient civilizations preserved meats, fish, and vegetables using salt for centuries. It draws out moisture, creating an environment where bacteria can't thrive. Use it in homemade pickles, cured meats, and brined vegetables. It's the classic preserver that stands the test of time.

5. Olive Oil: The Liquid Shield

- Olive oil can function as a protective barrier for cheeses, meats, and even fresh herbs. Drizzle it over salads, use it in marinades, or store your herbs in it to extend their shelf life. It's the liquid shield that adds flavor and freshness.

6. Homemade Ketchup: The Condiment Revolution

- It is common for store-bought ketchup to be loaded with sugar and preservatives. Make your own with tomatoes, vinegar, honey, and a blend of spices. Simmer until thick, blend until smooth, and enjoy a healthier, tastier version of this classic condiment. It's a condiment revolution in a bottle.

7. DIY Pickles: The Crisp Craze

- Skip the store-bought pickles and make your own with cucumbers, vinegar, garlic, dill, and a pinch of salt. Let them sit in the fridge for a few days, and you'll have crunchy, flavorful pickles without the artificial additives. It's the crisp craze that's easy and satisfying.

8. Natural Fruit Preserves: The Sweet Simplicity

- Instead of reaching for jam filled with high-fructose corn syrup, make your own fruit preserves. Use fresh fruit, a bit of honey or maple syrup, and a splash of lemon juice. Simmer until thickened, and you've got a jar of sweet simplicity ready to spread on toast or swirl into yogurt.

9. Herbal Teas: The Soothing Sip

- Ditch the store-bought tea bags and blend your own herbal teas using dried herbs like chamomile, peppermint, and hibiscus. Store them in airtight containers, and you'll have a soothing, preservative-free sip whenever you need it. It's the DIY tea time that's calming and creative.

10. Fresh Salsa: The Zesty Fiesta

- Forget jarred salsa and whip up a fresh batch with tomatoes, onions, cilantro, lime juice, and a pinch of salt. It's perfect for dipping, topping, or just eating with a spoon. It's a zesty fiesta in every bite.

11. Natural Yogurt: The Creamy Delight

- Make your yogurt with just milk and a bit of starter culture. It's easy, delicious, and free from artificial thickeners and sweeteners. Add fresh fruit or honey for a creamy delight that's as good for your gut as it is for your taste buds.

12. Homemade Bread: The Fresh Loaf

- Bake your bread with whole grain flour, yeast, water, and a pinch of salt. Skip the preservatives and enjoy the aroma of fresh-baked bread wafting through your kitchen. It's the fresh loaf that's wholesome and heartwarming.

In summary, using natural preservatives and making homemade versions of common foods is a delightful and healthful way to enjoy your meals. With a little creativity and some basic ingredients, you can transform your kitchen into a haven of natural goodness. Prepare yourself to appreciate the charm of homemade and naturally preserved foods by getting involved! Stay creative, stay healthy, and let nature's goodness shine in your kitchen, my friend!

Case Studies-Personal Account: Story of Someone Who Cut Out Artificial Additives from Their Diet

Meet Emily, a 38-year-old graphic designer with a flair for creativity and a love for all things tasty. Her diet was a colorful array of processed snacks, instant meals, and sugary drinks—each brimming with artificial additives and preservatives. Emily never gave much thought to what was in her food until she started experiencing frequent headaches, digestive issues, and an overall sense of fatigue.

One day, Emily stumbled upon an article about the potential health risks of artificial additives. Intrigued and a bit alarmed, she decided it was time to make a change. She embarked on a mission to cut out artificial additives from her diet and see if it could improve her well-being.

The first step was a daunting one—Emily had to purge her pantry. Out went the neon-colored cereals, the instant noodles with ingredient lists longer than a novel, and the sugary sodas. In their place, she stocked up on fresh fruits, vegetables, whole grains, and lean proteins. Her kitchen transformed from a processed food haven to a shrine of natural goodness.

Emily quickly realized that eating additive-free required a bit more effort, but she was up for the challenge. She began cooking more at home, experimenting with new recipes and flavors. Breakfasts became a joy with homemade granola and fresh fruit smoothies. Lunches featured colorful salads with a rainbow of veggies and homemade dressings. Dinners turned into creative culinary projects, with dishes like lemon herb chicken and roasted vegetables.

Within a few weeks, Emily started noticing changes. Her headaches became less frequent, her digestion improved, and she felt more energetic than she had in years. She even dropped a few pounds, not from dieting, but simply from eating whole, unprocessed foods.

But it wasn't just the physical changes that Emily experienced. Her mood improved, and she felt more balanced and less stressed. She discovered a newfound love for cooking and found it therapeutic to create meals from scratch. Her friends and family noticed her glow and asked her for tips on eating healthier.

Emily's journey wasn't without its challenges. She missed the convenience of processed foods, especially during busy workdays. But she learned to meal prep on weekends, making large batches of homemade soups, stews, and snacks that she could grab on the go. She also became a pro at reading labels, avoiding anything with unpronounceable ingredients or numbers.

One of the most rewarding moments for Emily was when she hosted a dinner party and served an entirely additive-free meal. The delicious and satisfying taste of the food amazed her guests, and some even changed their diets. Emily had become a beacon of inspiration, showing that cutting out artificial additives didn't mean sacrificing flavor or enjoyment.

Today, Emily is healthier and happier than ever. She continues to embrace a diet free from artificial additives and enjoys sharing her journey with others. Her story is a testament to the power of natural, whole foods and the incredible impact they can have on our health and well-being.

In conclusion, Emily's account highlights the benefits of cutting out artificial additives and embracing a diet of natural, wholesome foods. Her journey is an inspiring example of how minor changes can lead to significant improvements in health and happiness.

Embrace the journey, stay inspired, and let Emily's story motivate you to explore the world of additive-free living!

Personal Account: The Perils of Food Colorings

Meet Karen, a well-meaning mother of an energetic 8-year-old boy named Tommy. Karen loved to make Tommy's meals colorful and fun. Karen made vibrant bowls of neon-colored cereals for his breakfasts, packed lunches with rainbow-colored gummy snacks, and often served bright blue beverages and desserts covered in sprinkles for dinners.

Tommy's diet was a festival of artificial food colorings, and Karen took pride in her ability to make every meal a visual delight. But what Karen didn't realize was that those synthetic hues were more than just eye-catching—they were trouble brewing in a bowl.

As the weeks turned into months, Tommy's teachers began noticing some concerning changes. Tommy's teachers began noticing some concerning changes as the weeks turned into months. Tommy, who was once a focused and diligent student, now easily gets distracted, constantly fidgets, and often cannot sit still during lessons. He struggled to complete tasks, frequently interrupted the class, and seemed to be always in a state of restlessness.

At home, Tommy's behavior was no different. He had difficulty following instructions, threw tantrums over minor issues, and often clashed with his siblings. Karen attributed these changes to typical childhood antics, never suspecting that his diet might play a role.

A meeting with Tommy's teacher, Mrs. Thompson, brought the issue to the forefront. "Karen," Mrs. Thompson says gently, "we've observed significant behavioral changes in Tommy. Have you noticed anything similar at home?"

Karen nodded, perplexed. "Yes, he's been quite hyperactive and has trouble focusing."

Mrs. Thompson handed Karen a pamphlet. "There's growing evidence that artificial food colorings can contribute to attention deficit disorder (ADD) and other behavioral issues in children (Schab & Trinh, 2004). It might be worth considering his diet."

Karen's eyes widened in realization. Could it be? She went home and began researching. The information was overwhelming: studies linked synthetic food dyes like Red 40 and Yellow 5 to hyperactivity, ADD, and even developmental delays.

Determined to help her son, Karen overhauled Tommy's diet. Out went the colorful cereals, gummy snacks, and sugary drinks. She replaced them with whole foods, fresh fruits, and homemade meals free from artificial additives and dyes.

The transition was tough. Tommy missed his brightly colored treats and initially resisted the changes. But Karen persisted, knowing it was for his health and well-being. Slowly but surely, Tommy's behavior improved. He was calmer and more focused, and his tantrums decreased significantly.

But the story doesn't end there. Despite Karen's efforts, the years of high dye consumption had left their mark. Tommy continued to face challenges in school and social settings. His early exposure to these additives had set a hard path for his development.

One day, during a school field trip, a calamity struck. Tommy, overwhelmed and distracted, wandered off from the group. They searched frantically for hours before they found him, safe but shaken. The incident was a wake-up call for Karen and a stark reminder to other parents about the hidden dangers of artificial food colorings.

The ordeal served as a powerful lesson. Karen started a campaign at Tommy's school to raise awareness about the impact of food dyes on children's health. She shared her story at PTA meetings, urging other parents to reconsider the colorful but harmful additives in their children's diets.

In conclusion, Karen's story is a cautionary tale about the perils of inundating children with artificial food colorings. The link between these dyes and ADD, behavioral issues, and developmental problems is a serious concern. Let Tommy's experience be a lesson: choose natural, wholesome foods for your children and avoid the colorful traps that could lead to unforeseen consequences. Stay mindful, stay informed, and protect your children's health!

Ingredient 7: High Fructose Corn Syrup: The "Merchant of Death Found Everywhere"

What is HFCS?

Production Process and Why It's Used in So Many Foods

Sweet-toothed sleuths, it's time to delve into the sticky, syrupy world of High-Fructose Corn Syrup (HFCS). This abundant sweetener has found its way into countless foods and beverages, but what exactly is it? How is it made, and why is it everywhere? Let's unravel the sugary saga of HFCS.

The Basics: What is HFCS?

- High-Fructose Corn Syrup is a sweetener made from cornstarch. It is like table sugar (sucrose) but contains a higher level of fructose. Unlike regular corn syrup, HFCS undergoes further processing to convert some of its glucose into fructose, creating a sweeter and more versatile product. It's like taking corn syrup to the next level on the sweetness scale.

The Production Process: From Corn to Syrup

1. **Corn Starch Extraction**: The journey begins with corn kernels, which are milled to extract corn starch.

2. **Conversion to Corn Syrup**: The corn starch is treated with enzymes to break it down into glucose, resulting in regular corn syrup.

3. **Fructose Formation**: Here's where the magic happens. Adding a second enzyme helps convert some of the glucose into fructose, creating a sweeter syrup. Typically, they adjust the level of fructose, resulting

in HFCS with either 42% or 55% fructose.

4. **Final Processing:** Then, we purify and blend the resulting syrup to the desired consistency, preparing it to sweeten a myriad of products.

Why It's Used: The Sweet Spot

- **Cost-Effective:** One of the main reasons HFCS is so prevalent is its cost. Made from corn, which is abundantly grown in the United States (mostly because of subsidies given by the Federal government to Corn farmers to grow corn), HFCS is cheaper than cane sugar. This cost-efficiency makes it an attractive option for food manufacturers looking to sweeten their products without breaking the bank.

- **Sweetness and Stability:** HFCS is sweeter than regular corn syrup and has a similar sweetness level to table sugar. Its high fructose content also helps keep moisture, ensuring that baked goods stay soft and chewy. It's like a sweet guardian keeping your snacks fresh.

- **Versatility:** HFCS blends easily into foods and beverages, enhancing flavor and texture. From soft drinks and sauces to baked goods and candies, its versatility knows no bounds. It's the chameleon of sweeteners, adapting to a variety of culinary needs.

- **Shelf-Life Extension:** The fructose in HFCS acts as a preservative, helping to extend the shelf life of products. This makes it a favorite for processed foods that need to stay fresh over long periods. It's like having a time-traveling sugar that keeps your snacks from going stale.

The Controversy: A Sticky Situation

- Despite its widespread use, HFCS has been the subject of much debate and controversy. Concerns about its potential links to obesity, diabetes, and other health issues have led many to question its safety. While science is still growing, many health experts recommend limiting intake of HFCS and other added sugars to promote better health.

In summary, High-Fructose Corn Syrup is a cost-effective, versatile sweetener made from corn. Its ability to enhance flavor, texture, and shelf life has made it a staple in the food industry. However, its health implications continue to spark debate, making it a sweetener worth understanding and consuming mindfully. Stay informed, stay healthy, and navigate the sweet world of HFCS with a discerning eye!

Health Risks: Links to Obesity, Diabetes, and Liver Disease

Alright, health crusaders, it's time to shine a spotlight on the dark side of High-Fructose Corn Syrup (HFCS). This ubiquitous sweetener might make our food taste delightful, but it comes with a heavy price tag for our health. Let's delve into the potential risks of HFCS and its links to obesity, diabetes, and liver disease.

Obesity: The Expanding Waistline

- Picture this: you're enjoying your favorite soda, unaware that the HFCS inside is sneakily working to expand your waistline. The body uses glucose for energy, while the liver metabolizes fructose and easily converts it to fat. Overconsumption of HFCS can lead to an increase in visceral fat, the notorious belly fat that surrounds your organs and contributes to that dreaded muffin top and what makes you gentlemen appear as if you are pregnant! It's like adding fuel to the fire of the obesity epidemic.

Diabetes: The Sugar Spike Strikes Again

- High-Fructose Corn Syrup can wreak havoc on your blood sugar levels. When you consume HFCS, it causes a rapid spike in blood sugar and insulin levels. Over time, this can lead to insulin resistance, a condition where your cells become less responsive to insulin. This resistance forces your pancreas to produce more insulin to keep blood sugar levels in check, eventually leading to type 2 diabetes. It's like your body's sugar control system going haywire, with HFCS as the mischievous culprit.

Liver Disease: The Hidden Hazard

- The liver is the primary organ responsible for metabolizing fructose, and too much HFCS can overwhelm it. Excessive intake of HFCS can lead to the accumulation of fat in the liver, a condition known as non-alcoholic fatty liver disease (NAFLD) (Mizel, 2023). If left unchecked, NAFLD can progress to more severe liver conditions, such as non-alcoholic steatohepatitis (NASH), liver fibrosis, and even cirrhosis. It's like your liver turning into a storage unit for unwanted fat, with serious health consequences.

The Domino Effect: Other Health Concerns

- Besides obesity, diabetes, and liver disease, researchers have linked HFCS consumption to other health issues, such as increased triglycerides, which can raise the risk of heart disease (Hyman, 2014) (Lustig, 2012) (Taubes, 2016). It's like a domino effect of health problems, each tipping the next over, starting with a sweetened treat.

The Bigger Picture: Dietary Impact

- HFCS is present in a plethora of processed foods, such as sodas and fruit juices, candies, cereals, and baked goods. Its prevalence in the modern diet makes it easy to consume more than you realize. Reducing HFCS intake involves being mindful of food choices and opting for whole, unprocessed foods. It's about reclaiming control over your diet and making healthier choices.

In conclusion, while HFCS adds sweetness to our favorite foods and beverages, its health risks are too significant to ignore. Links to obesity, diabetes, and liver disease highlight the need for caution and moderation. By being aware of high fructose corn syrup in your diet, you can take proactive measures to safeguard your health and well-being. Stay vigilant, stay healthy, and keep those sugary culprits in check, my beloved reader friend!

Countries with Restrictions or Bans on HFCS

1. European Union (EU):

While not technically banned in the EU, HFCS faces heavy regulation under names such as "glucose-fructose syrup" or "fructose-glucose syrup." Quotas on production and use of HFCS have reduced consumption to levels well below that of the U.S.. The application of this expanding regulation approaches a passive view on the universal use of HFCS in food products.

2. Japan:

Import quotas and high tariffs in Japan constrain the use of HFCS. Japan is a country that prefers the use of natural sweeteners such as sugar, stevia, and rice syrup, translating to lower HFCS consumption in the Japanese diet.

3. Mexico:

Mexico, meanwhile, has previously hit U.S. HFCS with import tariffs to shield its large sugar industry from competition. The greater popularity of cane sugar and a history of fluctuating tariffs have led to substantial opposition to extensive use by HFCS.

Global Perspectives on Health

1. Health Concerns:

The correlation of HFCS with obesity, type 2 diabetes, and liver disease and some health-related risks detected by this study are enormous. This is because HFCS contains a much higher fructose content than glucose, and our body metabolizes fructose differently. Ingesting high levels of fructose can cause metabolic problems, which is why it poses health-related risks.

2. Public Sentiment and Market Demand:

Several nations have steered towards natural and less processed food. This trend has reduced the consumption of HFCS, while increasing demand for these natural sweeteners like honey, maple syrup, & cane sugar. Consumer perception shapes the formation of broader food industry practices and regulatory policies.

3. Industry Adaptations:

In these regions, many food products produced by major manufacturers contain high-fructose corn syrup to reduce expenses and withstand the regulatory and consumer-driven shifts in the legal system. Perhaps most importantly, this re-interpretation shows a larger movement towards cleaner substitutions overall in the category.

Conclusion

While HFCS is not banned outright, different countries place various restrictions (e.g., import tariffs) and regulations on it. These steps show mounting health concerns and a worldwide pattern towards healthier groceries with fewer carbs. This broader way of thinking about these issues may help us understand a little more why it is crucial to make healthy choices and support public policies that work towards making our food system healthier for all concerned.

Avoiding HFCS: Foods to Watch Out for and How to Choose HFCS-Free Products

Alright, savvy shoppers and health enthusiasts, it's time to embark on a quest to dodge the lurking HFCS in our food. This sneaky sweetener hides in places you'd least expect, but with a bit of knowledge and vigilance, you can keep it off your plate. Let's dive into the foods to watch out for and tips on choosing HFCS-free products.

Foods to Watch Out For: The Usual Suspects

1. Sodas and Soft Drinks: The Fizzing Foes

- Sodas are the poster children for HFCS. That fizzy, sweet beverage often contains this syrupy sweetener. If it's bubbly and sugary, it's likely harboring HFCS. Opt for sparkling water or homemade infused water instead.

2. Sweetened Fruit Juices: The Deceptive Drinks

- Fruit juices, especially those labeled as "fruit drinks" or "cocktails," are notorious for containing HFCS. Even some "natural" fruit juices can have added HFCS. Choose 100% fruit juice or, better yet, squeeze your own.

3. Snacks and Baked Goods: The Tempting Traps

- Cookies, cakes, muffins, and snack bars often contain HFCS to keep them moist and sweet. Check the ingredient list on your favorite treats and look for brands that use natural sweeteners instead.

4. Breakfast Cereals: The Morning Mischief

- Many popular breakfast cereals, especially those marketed to children, commonly contain HFCS. Look for cereals with short ingredient lists and sweetened

109

with natural options like honey or dried fruit.

5. Condiments: The Sneaky Saucers

- Ketchup, barbecue sauce, salad dressings, and even some mustards can be HFCS hotbeds. Opt for condiments labeled "no high-fructose corn syrup" or make your own at home for a healthier alternative.

6. Processed Snacks: The Crunchy Culprits

- Chips, crackers, and other processed snacks often contain HFCS. Choose whole grain or baked versions and check the ingredient list for any hidden sweeteners.

7. Canned and Packaged Foods: The Hidden Hazards

- HFCS can lurk in canned soups, packaged meals, and even some savory items like baked beans. Always read the labels to ensure you're not getting an unexpected dose of HFCS.

How to Choose HFCS-Free Products: The Smart Shopper's Guide

1. Read Labels: The Detective's Delight

- Become a label-reading specialist. Ingredients are listed in descending order by weight, meaning the most abundant are at the top, so if HFCS is near the top, it's a major component. Look for products with short, recognizable ingredient lists.

2. Look for Certifications: The Trusty Badges

- Products labeled "organic" or "non-GMO" are less likely to contain HFCS. These certifications can help guide you toward healthier choices.

3. Choose Whole Foods: The Natural Way

- Choose whole, unprocessed foods. Fresh fruits, vegetables, whole grains, and lean proteins are naturally HFCS-free. It's the easiest way to avoid hidden sweeteners.

4. Shop the Perimeter: The Outer Ring Rule

- The perimeter of the grocery store is where you'll find fresh produce, dairy, and meats—foods that are typically free from HFCS. The inner aisles are where processed foods and hidden sweeteners lurk.

5. DIY: The Homemade Hero

- Making snacks, baked goods, and condiments allows you to control the ingredients and avoid HFCS altogether. Plus, it's a fun and rewarding way to experiment in the kitchen.

6. Ask Questions: The Curious Consumer

- Don't be afraid to ask questions at restaurants or when shopping. Many places are happy to provide information about their ingredients. Knowledge plus action is power, and it's your right to know what you're consuming.

7. Stay Informed: The Knowledge Seeker

- Keep up with the latest information on HFCS and other food additives. Being informed helps you make better choices for yourself and your family.

In summary, avoiding HFCS involves being vigilant and informed about the foods you consume. By reading labels, choosing whole foods, and making your meals, you can steer clear of this sneaky sweetener and enjoy a healthier diet. Happy shopping and may your journey to HFCS-free living be sweet in all the right ways! Stay savvy, stay informed, and keep HFCS off your plate.

Dietary Changes: Tips for Eliminating HFCS and Healthier

Sweetening Options

Alright, sugar investigators, it's time to banish High-Fructose Corn Syrup (HFCS) from your diet and embrace healthier, more natural sweetening options. With a few simple changes and a bit of culinary creativity, you can enjoy deliciously sweet foods without the health risks. Let's dive into some tips for eliminating HFCS and discovering healthier alternatives.

1. Clean Out the Pantry: The Great HFCS Purge

- Start by purging your pantry of HFCS-laden foods. Toss out those neon-colored cereals, sugary sodas, processed snacks, and canned goods with hidden HFCS. It's time for a fresh start with a pantry stocked with wholesome, HFCS-free goodies.

2. Become a Label Detective: The Ingredient Investigator

- Get into the habit of reading labels like a pro. Look for HFCS and its aliases (like glucose-fructose syrup) in the ingredient lists. Choose products with simple, recognizable ingredients and avoid those with long lists of unpronounceable additives.

3. Go for Whole Foods: The Natural Choice

- Whole foods like fruits, vegetables, whole grains, nuts, and seeds are naturally free from HFCS. Make these the foundation of your diet. They're not only healthier but also packed with essential nutrients and fiber.

4. Cook at Home: The DIY Delight

- When you cook at home, you control what goes into your food. Experiment with homemade versions of your favorite dishes and snacks. It's a fun and rewarding way to ensure you're eating HFCS-free meals.

5. Choose Natural Sweeteners: The Healthier Alternatives

- Replace HFCS with natural sweeteners that add flavor and nutrition to your foods. Here are some great options:
  - **Honey**: A natural sweetener with antibacterial properties. Perfect for tea, yogurt, and baking.
  - **Maple Syrup**: Rich in antioxidants and minerals, ideal for pancakes, waffles, and even savory dishes.
  - **Agave Nectar**: A low-glycemic sweetener great for smoothies, oatmeal, and desserts.
  - **Stevia**: A calorie-free sweetener derived from the stevia plant. Use it in beverages and baking for a guilt-free sweet fix.
  - **Coconut Sugar**: A low-glycemic sweetener with a caramel-like flavor. Use it in baking, sauces, and coffee.

6. Swap Sugary Drinks: The Refreshing Change

- Ditch the sodas and sugary fruit drinks. Pick water, herbal teas, or homemade infused waters with fresh fruits and herbs. Sparkling water with a splash of fruit juice is also a great HFCS-free alternative.

7. Snack Smart: The Wholesome Munchies

- Choose snacks that are naturally sweet and satisfying. Fresh fruit, nuts, seeds, and homemade granola bars are excellent choices. They'll keep you energized without the HFCS overload.

8. Enjoy Naturally Sweetened Treats: The Sweet Swap

- When a sweet craving strikes, reach for treats sweetened with natural ingredients. Make your own cookies, muffins, and cakes using honey, maple syrup, or ripe bananas. You'll get all the sweetness without the health risks.

9. Educate Yourself: The Knowledge is Power

- Stay informed about the foods you eat and the ingredients they contain. Follow health blogs, read nutrition labels, and keep up with the latest research on sweeteners and additives. The more you know, the better choices you can make.

10. Spread the Word: The Sweet Advocate

- Share your journey with friends and family. Encourage them to join you in eliminating HFCS and making healthier choices. The more people are aware of the risks of HFCS, the greater the collective effort to avoid it.

In summary, eliminating HFCS from your diet involves making informed choices, cooking at home, and opting for natural sweeteners. With these tips, you can enjoy the sweetness in your life without compromising your health. So embark on your HFCS-free journey and savor the delicious, wholesome flavors that nature offers. Stay sweet, stay healthy, and enjoy your HFCS-free lifestyle.

Case Study-Transformation Story: Individual Who Eliminated HFCS and Experienced Significant Health Improvements

Meet Samantha, a 42-year-old marketing executive who juggled a hectic work schedule with raising two teenagers. Samantha's life was a whirlwind of meetings, deadlines, and fast-food meals. Her diet was a collage of convenience foods —sugary sodas, instant noodles, and pre-packaged snacks, all laden with High-Fructose Corn Syrup (HFCS).

Samantha thought little about her diet until she started

noticing some unwelcome changes. She constantly felt fatigued, struggled to concentrate, and gained extra pounds that refused to go away. Frequent headaches and digestive issues became her new normal. After a particularly stressful week, Samantha decided it was time to take control of her health.

One evening, she stumbled upon an old classmate who talked to her about the health risks of HFCS, including its links to obesity, diabetes, and liver disease. The talk was a wake-up call. Determined to make a change, Samantha embarked on a mission to eliminate HFCS from her diet.

The first step was a kitchen overhaul. Samantha purged her pantry of all HFCS-laden foods—goodbye neon-colored cereals, sugary drinks, and processed snacks. She replaced them with fresh fruits, vegetables, whole grains, and lean proteins. Her kitchen transformed from a convenience store into a sanctuary of wholesome, natural foods.

Samantha quickly discovered that eliminating HFCS required more than just a pantry purge; it required vigilance. She became addicted to label-reading scanning ingredient lists for hidden HFCS and choosing products with simple, recognizable ingredients. Her grocery shopping trips became a quest for natural and organic options.

Breakfasts were the first to change. Instead of sugary cereals, Samantha enjoyed Greek yogurt with fresh berries and a drizzle of honey. Lunches became vibrant salads with a rainbow of veggies and homemade dressings. Dinners turned into creative culinary projects, with dishes like baked salmon with quinoa and roasted vegetables.

As the weeks passed, Samantha noticed remarkable changes. Her energy levels soared, and the constant fatigue vanished. She could focus better at work, and her productivity improved. The extra pounds melted away, and her clothes fit better. Even her skin cleared up, giving her a healthy glow.

But the benefits didn't stop there. Samantha's headaches

became less frequent, and her digestive issues improved dramatically. She felt more balanced, both physically and mentally. Her family noticed the positive changes and joined her on the HFCS-free journey.

Samantha's transformation didn't go unnoticed at work. Her colleagues admired her newfound energy and enthusiasm. She became an advocate for healthy eating, sharing her story and tips with anyone who would listen. Her dedication inspired others to reconsider their own diets and make healthier choices.

One day, Samantha saw her doctor for a check-up. The results were astonishing. Her blood sugar levels were stable, her cholesterol had improved, and her liver function was better than ever. The doctor was amazed at the transformation and motivated her to continue doing great. He commented that even when he was in medical school; he learned very little about the impact and importance of nutrition.

Samantha's journey wasn't without its challenges. She missed the convenience of processed foods, especially during busy days. But she learned to meal prep on weekends, making large batches of homemade soups, stews, and snacks that she could grab on the go. She also discovered a love for cooking and found it therapeutic to create meals from scratch.

Today, Samantha is a testament to the power of eliminating HFCS from one's diet. She's healthier, happier, and more vibrant than ever. Her story is a shining example of how minor dietary changes can lead to significant health improvements. By cutting out HFCS, Samantha reclaimed her health and her zest for life.

In conclusion, Samantha's transformation story highlights the incredible benefits of eliminating HFCS and embracing a diet of natural, wholesome foods. Her journey is an inspiring example of how making mindful choices can lead to a healthier, happier life. Stay inspired, stay healthy, and let Samantha's story motivate you to take control of your diet and health, my friend!

CONCLUSION

Recap of Key Points:

*Summary of the Main Takeaways
from Each Chapter*

Chapter 1: Refined Sugars

- **Key Takeaways**: We explored the sweet yet sinister world of refined sugars, delving into their prevalence in our diets and their addictive nature. Excessive consumption leads to obesity, diabetes, and heart disease, making it crucial to cut back. Hidden sources of sugar, like salad dressings and bread, taught us to read labels like detectives to uncover these sneaky sugars.

- **My Top Suggestion**: Replace sugary beverages with water or herbal tea. This simple switch can drastically reduce your sugar intake and improve your overall health.

Chapter 2: Trans Fats

- **Key Takeaways**: Trans fats are the villains of the fat world, lurking in fried foods and baked goods. They raise bad cholesterol and lower good cholesterol, significantly increasing the risk of heart disease. Healthier cooking methods, like baking and grilling, can help us avoid these harmful fats and protect our hearts.

- **My Top Suggestion**: Avoid processed foods that list **"partially hydrogenated oils"** in the ingredients. Opt for foods with healthy fats like nuts, seeds, and avocados.

Chapter 3: Saturated Fats

- **Key Takeaways**: Red meat, butter, and cheese contain saturated fats, which add flavor but also clog arteries and increase the risk of cardiovascular disease. Moderation is key, and we learned to swap out saturated fats for healthier options like olive oil and avocados to keep our hearts happy.

- **My Top Suggestion**: Swap butter with olive oil or avocado in cooking and baking. This simple change can reduce your saturated fat intake and boost heart health.

Chapter 4: Refined Carbohydrates

- **Key Takeaways**: Refined carbohydrates, such as white bread, pastries, and sugary cereals, spike blood sugar levels and contribute to obesity and type 2 diabetes. Switching to whole grains and fiber-rich foods helps maintain stable energy levels and supports overall health.

- **My Top Suggestion**: Replace white bread and pasta with whole-grain versions. This swap provides more fiber and nutrients, helping you stay full and energized.

Chapter 5: High Sodium

- **Key Takeaways:** High sodium intake is linked to hypertension and cardiovascular diseases. Reading labels and choosing fresh, whole foods is crucial because processed foods often contain hidden sodium. We discussed strategies for reducing salt in our diets, such as using herbs and spices for flavor.

- **My Top Suggestion**: Season your meals with herbs and spices instead of salt. This enhances flavor without the added sodium.

Chapter 6: Artificial Additives and Preservatives

- **Key Takeaways**: Artificial additives and preservatives, including synthetic food dyes and flavor enhancers, can cause a range of health issues from hyperactivity in children to digestive problems and allergic reactions. Choosing natural alternatives and making homemade versions of common foods helps avoid these harmful ingredients.

- **My Top Suggestion**: Choose products with short,

recognizable ingredient lists. The fewer the ingredients, the better, and aim for those you can pronounce.

Chapter 7: High-Fructose Corn Syrup (HFCS)

- **Key Takeaways**: HFCS is a cheap and pervasive sweetener linked to obesity, diabetes, and liver disease. Eliminating HFCS involves reading labels, avoiding processed foods, and opting for natural sweeteners like honey and maple syrup. The benefits of cutting out HFCS include better energy levels, weight loss, and improved overall health.

- **My Top Suggestion**: Replace soda and fruit drinks with water infused with fresh fruit. This helps you avoid HFCS while enjoying a refreshing, naturally sweet beverage.

The Power of Choice: Take Control of Your Health Through Informed Food Choices

Alright, health warriors, it's time to embrace the power of choice and take the reins of your well-being. In a world where convenience often trumps nutrition, making informed food choices is your secret weapon to achieve vibrant health and longevity. Let's delve into why taking control of your diet is the ultimate act of self-care and empowerment.

Empowerment Through Knowledge

- Knowledge is power, and in your diet, it's the key to unlocking a healthier you. By understanding what goes into your food and how it affects your body, you can make choices that support your well-being. Say goodbye to blindly consuming what's convenient and hello to being a savvy, informed eater. You can do this!

Reading Labels: The Detective Work

- Imagine yourself as a food detective, scanning labels with the precision of Sherlock Holmes. By deciphering ingredient lists and nutritional information, you can uncover hidden sugars, unhealthy fats, and artificial additives. This detective work empowers you to choose products that nourish your body instead of weighing it down with harmful substances.

Choosing Whole Foods: The Natural Advantage

- Whole foods like fruits, vegetables, whole grains, and lean proteins are your allies in the quest for better health. These foods contain essential nutrients, fiber, and natural goodness that processed foods simply can't match. By filling your plate with whole foods, you're making a powerful choice to fuel your body with what it truly needs.

Cooking at Home: The Culinary Revolution

- When you cook at home, you're in the driver's seat. You control the ingredients, the preparation, and the portion sizes. This not only helps you avoid hidden additives and excess calories but also allows you to experiment with flavors and create meals you love. Plus, it's a fun and rewarding way to connect with your food. The major issue with this is that you have to be certain that the food you purchase is from a clean, preferably organic, non-GMO source.

Mindful Eating: The Conscious Connection

- Mindful eating is all about being present and fully experiencing your meals. By paying attention to what you eat, savoring each bite, and listening to your body's hunger and fullness cues, you can build a healthier relationship with food. It's not just about what you eat, but how you eat it.

Small Changes, Big Impact

- Remember, you don't have to overhaul your diet

overnight. Small, gradual changes can lead to significant improvements in your health. Start by making one healthier choice at a time—swap sugary drinks with water, choose whole grain bread over white, or snack on fresh fruit instead of candy. Each small step brings you closer to your health goals.

Inspiring Others: The Ripple Effect

- Your journey towards healthier eating doesn't just benefit you; it can inspire those around you. By making informed food choices, you set a positive example for your friends, family, and community. Together, we can create a ripple effect on health and wellness.

In conclusion, the power of choice is in your hands. By making informed decisions about what you eat, you can take control of your health and transform your life. Embrace your inner food detective, fill your plate with whole foods, and savor the journey to better well-being. You have the power to choose health, happiness, and vitality—so make it happen!

Next Steps: Practical Advice for Implementing the Changes Suggested in the Book

Alright, health crusaders, you've armed yourself with knowledge of the seven deadly ingredients. Now it's time to put that knowledge into action and transform your diet. Here are some practical, down-to-earth steps to help you implement the changes suggested in the book and embark on your journey to better health:

1. Clean Out Your Pantry: The Great Detox

- Start by purging your pantry and fridge of foods that contain refined sugars, trans fats, high sodium, artificial additives, and HFCS. Donate unopened items to a local food bank if possible. Fill the empty spaces with wholesome, natural foods like fresh fruits, vegetables, whole grains, nuts, and lean proteins. It's like spring cleaning for your health!

2. Become a Label Detective: Read Before You Buy

- Make it a habit to read food labels every time you shop. Look out for those sneaky ingredients you want to avoid, such as "high-fructose corn syrup," "partially hydrogenated oils," and any unpronounceable additives. If the ingredient list reads like a chemistry exam, put it back on the shelf. You've got the power to choose better options.

3. Cook at Home: Master Your Kitchen

- Take control of what goes into your meals by cooking at home more often. Not a seasoned chef? No worries! Start with simple recipes and gradually try more complex dishes as you gain confidence. Batch cooking and meal prepping can save time and ensure you have healthy meals ready to go during busy weeks. Your kitchen is your kingdom—rule it wisely!

4. Plan Your Meals: The Blueprint for Success

- Planning your meals ahead of time can help you stay on track and avoid impulse buys. Create a weekly meal plan that includes a variety of whole foods and balanced meals. Make a shopping list based on your plan and stick to it when you go grocery shopping. Planning is your secret weapon against the lure of convenience foods.

5. Swap Smartly: Easy Substitutions

- Replace refined and processed ingredients with healthier alternatives. For example, use whole grain bread instead of white bread, olive oil instead of butter, and fresh fruit instead of sugary snacks. These small swaps can make a big difference in your overall diet. It's all about upgrading your choices.

6. Hydrate Wisely: Drink to Your Health

- Ditch sugary sodas and fruit drinks. Instead, hydrate with water, herbal teas, and homemade infused waters. Add slices of lemon, cucumber, or berries to your water for a refreshing twist. Staying hydrated supports your body's functions and helps you feel energized.

7. Snack Smart: Keep It Simple

- Keep healthy snacks on hand to avoid the temptation of junk food. Fresh fruits, nuts, seeds, and homemade granola bars are excellent choices. Prepare snack packs ahead of time so you have something healthy to grab when hunger strikes. Snacking smart keeps you satisfied and on track.

8. Educate Yourself: Stay Informed

- Continue learning about nutrition and healthy eating. Follow health blogs, read books, and stay updated on the latest research. Knowledge and action is power, and the more you know, the better choices (actions) you can make. Make it a lifelong commitment to stay informed and empowered.

9. Join a community: Support and Share

- Connect with others who are on the same journey. Join a local health club, cooking class, or online community where you can share tips, recipes, and support. Having a community can keep you motivated and accountable. Together, you can celebrate successes and overcome challenges.

10. Be Patient and Persistent: Progress, Not Perfection

- Remember, change takes time. Be patient with yourself and celebrate small victories along the way. It's not about perfection, but about making progress. Every step you take towards healthier eating is a step in the right direction. Stay persistent, and do not let setbacks discourage you. You've got this!

In conclusion, implementing these changes is a journey, not a sprint. By taking practical steps, staying informed, and being patient, you can transform your diet and improve your health. Embrace the power of choice, and enjoy the journey to a healthier, happier you!

Resources: Further Reading, Helpful Websites, and Tools for Continued Learning

Listen, knowledge seekers, the journey to better health doesn't end at a spot. It is a continuous process. To help you stay informed and empowered, I have compiled a list of invaluable resources. Dive into these books, explore these websites, and use these tools to continue your quest for a healthier lifestyle.

Must-Read Books

1. **"The Omnivore's Dilemma," by Michael Pollan:**
   - Explore the complexities of our food choices and the impact they have on our health and the environment. Pollan's investigative journey through the food chain is eye-opening and engaging.

2. **"Salt Sugar Fat: How the Food Giants Hooked Us," by Michael Moss:**
   - Discover the inside story of how big food companies have manipulated our cravings with addictive ingredients. Moss's exposé is both shocking and enlightening.

3. **"In Defense of Food: An Eater's Manifesto," by Michael Pollan:**
   - Pollan returns with a simple yet profound message: "Eat food. Not too much. Mostly plants." This book offers practical advice for making healthier food choices.

4. **"The Whole30: The 30-Day Guide to Total Health and Food Freedom," by Melissa Hartwig Urban and Dallas Hartwig:**
   - This book provides a comprehensive guide to eliminating harmful foods from your diet and discovering a healthier, more balanced way of eating.

Helpful Websites: Go To Online Resources

1. **Fooducate (www.fooducate.com):**
   - An excellent tool for deciphering food labels and making healthier choices. Fooducate offers product reviews, nutritional information, and a helpful app for on-the-go decisions.

2. **Environmental Working Group (EWG) (www.ewg.org):**
   - EWG's website is a treasure trove of information on food safety, additives, and healthy living. Check out their guides on pesticides in produce and their food scores database.

3. **The Center for Science in the Public Interest (CSPI) (www.cspinet.org):**
   - CSPI provides reliable, science-based information on nutrition and health. Their resources include articles, reports, and tips for healthier eating.

4. **Harvard T.H. Chan School of Public Health (www.hsph.harvard.edu/nutritionsource):**
   - A comprehensive resource for evidence-based nutrition information. Explore their guides on various dietary topics, including fats, carbohydrates, and sodium.

Tools for Continued Learning: Apps and Online Courses

1. **MyFitnessPal:**
   - This popular app helps you track your food intake, exercise, and nutritional goals. It's a great tool for staying accountable and making informed choices.

2. **Yummly:**
   - Yummly offers personalized recipe recommendations based on your dietary preferences. It's perfect for discovering new, healthy meals to try at home.

3. **Coursera:**
   - Coursera offers online courses from top universities on nutrition and health. Enroll in courses like "The Science of Well-Being" by Yale University or "Nutrition and Lifestyle in Pregnancy" by Ludwig Maximilian University of Munich.

4. **Udemy:**
   - Udemy has a variety of courses on healthy cooking, meal planning, and nutrition. Whether you're a beginner or looking to expand your knowledge, there's a course for you.

Community Support: Finding Your Tribe

1. **Meetup (www.meetup.com):**
   - Find local groups focused on healthy eating, cooking, and fitness. Join meetups to connect with like-minded individuals and share your journey.

2. **Reddit (www.reddit.com):**
   - Subreddits like r/nutrition, r/healthyfood, and r/Whole30 offer communities of

support, advice, and inspiration. Engage in discussions, ask questions, and learn from others' experiences.

3. **Facebook Groups**:
    ◦ Join Facebook groups dedicated to healthy eating and lifestyle changes. Look for groups focused on specific diets, such as Paleo, Whole30, or plant-based living.

4. **Instagram**:
    ◦ Follow health-focused accounts and hashtags like #healthyeating, #cleaneating, and #nutrition. Engage with the community, share your journey, and find daily inspiration from others on a similar path.

5. **Twitter**:
    ◦ Follow nutrition experts, health organizations, and fitness influencers. Take part in Twitter chats on health topics, share your progress, and stay updated on the latest health trends with hashtags like #HealthyLiving and #Nutrition.

In conclusion, the journey to better health is ongoing, and these resources will keep you informed, inspired, and empowered. Dive into the books, explore the websites, and use the tools and communities available to you. Your quest for a healthier lifestyle is a lifelong adventure—embrace it with curiosity and enthusiasm!

In addition, browse the "Works Cited" pages of this book for further information and resources

APPENDIX

Recipes:

Collection of Healthy Recipes Free from the Seven Deadly Ingredients

Here we go, culinary adventurers, it's time to embark on a delicious journey with two days of recipes that are free from refined sugars, trans fats, saturated fats, refined carbohydrates, high sodium, artificial additives and preservatives, and high-fructose corn syrup. These recipes are not only healthy but also bursting with flavor. Let's get cooking!

1. Breakfast: Avocado and Spinach Smoothie

Ingredients:

- 1 ripe avocado
- 1 cup fresh spinach leaves
- 1 banana
- 1 cup unsweetened almond milk
- 1 tablespoon chia seeds
- 1 teaspoon honey (optional)
- Ice cubes (optional)

Instructions:

1. Cut the avocado in half, remove the pit, and scoop the flesh into a blender.
2. Add the spinach, banana, almond milk, and chia

seeds.

3. Blend until smooth. If you prefer a colder smoothie, add ice cubes and blend again.

4. Taste and add honey if you like it sweeter.

5. Pour into a glass and enjoy a nutrient-packed start to your day!

2. Lunch: Quinoa and Black Bean Salad

Ingredients:

- 1 cup quinoa, rinsed
- 2 cups water
- 1 can black beans, rinsed and drained
- 1 red bell pepper, diced
- 1 cucumber, diced
- 1/4 cup red onion, finely chopped
- 1/4 cup fresh cilantro, chopped
- 1 avocado, diced
- Juice of 2 limes
- 2 tablespoons olive oil
- 1 teaspoon ground cumin
- Black pepper to taste

Instructions:

1. In a medium saucepan, bring the quinoa and water to a boil. Reduce heat, cover, and simmer for 15 minutes or until the water is absorbed. Let cool.

2. In a large bowl, combine the cooked quinoa, black beans, bell pepper, cucumber, red onion, and cilantro.

3. In a small bowl, whisk together the lime juice, olive oil, cumin, and black pepper.

4. Pour the dressing over the salad and toss to combine.

5. Gently fold in the diced avocado.

6. Serve chilled and savor this refreshing, protein-packed salad.

3. Dinner: Baked Lemon Herb Salmon

Ingredients:

- 4 salmon filets
- 2 lemons (one sliced, one juiced)
- 3 cloves garlic, minced
- 2 tablespoons fresh parsley, chopped
- 1 tablespoon fresh dill, chopped
- 1 tablespoon olive oil
- Black pepper to taste

Instructions:

1. Preheat your oven to 375°F (190°C).

2. Place the salmon filets on a baking sheet lined with parchment paper.

3. In a small bowl, mix the lemon juice, garlic, parsley, dill, olive oil, and black pepper.

4. Spoon the mixture over the salmon filets.

5. Arrange lemon slices on top of the filets.

6. Bake for 20-25 minutes or until the salmon is cooked through and flakes easily with a fork.

7. Serve with a side of steamed vegetables or a fresh salad and enjoy a delicious, heart-healthy meal.

4. Snack: Apple Slices with Almond Butter

Ingredients:

- 2 apples, cored and sliced

- 1/4 cup almond butter
- 1 tablespoon chia seeds
- 1 tablespoon unsweetened shredded coconut (optional)

Instructions:

1. Arrange the apple slices on a plate.
2. Dip or spread each slice with almond butter.
3. Sprinkle chia seeds and shredded coconut on top.
4. Enjoy this simple, satisfying snack that's free from refined sugars and full of healthy fats.

5. Dessert: Banana Oat Cookies

Ingredients:

- 2 ripe bananas, mashed
- 1 cup rolled oats
- 1/4 cup dark chocolate chips (optional, free from artificial additives)
- 1 teaspoon vanilla extract
- 1/2 teaspoon cinnamon

Instructions:

1. Preheat your oven to 350°F (175°C) and line a baking sheet with parchment paper.
2. In a large bowl, combine the mashed bananas, oats, chocolate chips, vanilla extract, and cinnamon.
3. Drop a spoonful of the dough onto the prepared baking sheet and flatten slightly with a fork.
4. Bake for 15 minutes or until the edges are golden brown.
5. Let cool on a wire rack and enjoy a healthy, naturally sweet treat.

In conclusion, these recipes provide delicious, wholesome alternatives to meals laden with the seven deadly ingredients. Enjoy creating and savoring these dishes, knowing they support your health and well-being.

Day 2 Recipes: Healthy and Delicious Meals Free from the Seven Deadly Ingredients

1. Breakfast: Berry Chia Pudding

Ingredients:

- 1 cup unsweetened almond milk
- 3 tablespoons chia seeds
- 1 cup mixed berries (fresh or frozen)
- 1 teaspoon vanilla extract
- 1 teaspoon honey (optional)

Instructions:

1. In a bowl, mix the almond milk, chia seeds, and vanilla extract.
2. Stir well, cover, and refrigerate for at least 4 hours or overnight.
3. Before serving, stir again and add the mixed berries on top.
4. Drizzle with honey if desired.
5. Enjoy a nutritious, fiber-rich start to your day!

2. Lunch: Mediterranean Chickpea Salad

Ingredients:

- 1 can chickpeas, rinsed and drained
- 1 cucumber, diced
- 1 cup cherry tomatoes, halved
- 1/4 red onion, finely chopped
- 1/4 cup Kalamata olives, sliced
- 1/4 cup feta cheese, crumbled (optional)

- 2 tablespoons olive oil
- Juice of 1 lemon
- 1 teaspoon dried oregano
- Black pepper to taste

Instructions:

1. In a large bowl, combine the chickpeas, cucumber, cherry tomatoes, red onion, and olives.

2. In a small bowl, whisk together the olive oil, lemon juice, oregano, and black pepper.

3. Pour the dressing over the salad and toss to combine.

4. Sprinkle with feta cheese if desired.

5. Serve chilled and enjoy the flavors of the Mediterranean.

3. Dinner: Stuffed Bell Peppers

Ingredients:

- 4 large bell peppers (any color), tops cut off and seeds removed
- 1 cup cooked quinoa
- 1 can black beans, rinsed and drained
- 1 cup corn kernels (fresh or frozen)
- 1 cup diced tomatoes
- 1/2 cup diced onion
- 2 cloves garlic, minced
- 1 tablespoon olive oil
- 1 teaspoon ground cumin
- 1 teaspoon smoked paprika
- Black pepper to taste
- 1/4 cup shredded cheese (optional)

Instructions:

1. Preheat your oven to 375°F (190°C).

2. In a large skillet, heat the olive oil over medium heat. Add the onion and garlic, and sauté until softened.

3. Stir in the quinoa, black beans, corn, diced tomatoes, cumin, smoked paprika, and black pepper. Cook for 5-7 minutes until heated through.

4. Place the bell peppers in a baking dish and stuff them with the quinoa mixture.

5. Sprinkle shredded cheese on top if desired.

6. Cover with foil and bake for 30 minutes. Remove the foil and bake for an additional 10 minutes.

7. Serve hot and enjoy a colorful, nutritious dinner.

4. Snack: Veggie Sticks with Hummus

Ingredients:

- 1 carrot, cut into sticks
- 1 cucumber, cut into sticks
- 1 bell pepper, cut into sticks
- 1 cup cherry tomatoes
- 1/2 cup hummus (homemade or store-bought without artificial additives)

Instructions:

1. Arrange the veggie sticks and cherry tomatoes on a plate.

2. Serve with a side of hummus for dipping.

3. Enjoy this crunchy, satisfying snack that's packed with vitamins and fiber.

5. Dessert: Coconut Mango

Energy Bites

Ingredients:

- 1 cup dried mango, chopped
- 1/2 cup shredded unsweetened coconut
- 1/2 cup almonds
- 1/4 cup chia seeds
- 2 tablespoons honey
- 1 teaspoon vanilla extract

Instructions:

1. In a food processor, combine the dried mango, shredded coconut, almonds, chia seeds, honey, and vanilla extract.
2. Pulse until the mixture is well combined and sticky.
3. Roll the mixture into small balls and place them on a baking sheet lined with parchment paper.
4. Refrigerate for at least 1 hour to set.
5. Enjoy these tropical energy bites as a healthy, naturally sweet treat.

In conclusion, these recipes provide another day of delicious, wholesome meals free from the seven deadly ingredients. Enjoy creating and savoring these dishes, knowing they support your health and well-being.

Shopping Guide: Navigating the 7 Deadly Ingredients

Purpose of the Guide

Welcome, intrepid health adventurers, to the ultimate shopping survival manual! This guide isn't just any old list of do's and don'ts—oh no, it's your trusty sidekick in the epic quest to banish the seven sinister, health-sabotaging ingredients lurking in your favorite foods. Imagine it as your culinary compass, pointing you away from dietary disaster and towards a land of vibrant health and vitality.

"Why?" you may ask. Well, dear reader, this guide aims to transform your grocery cart into a fortress of nutrition, fortified against the nefarious plots of refined sugars, trans fats, saturated fats, refined carbohydrates, high sodium, artificial additives, and that sneaky saboteur, high-fructose corn syrup (HFCS). We're here to help you decipher the hieroglyphics on ingredient labels, escape the pitfalls of processed foods, and emerge victorious in the battle for a healthier, happier you.

Picture this: You, striding confidently through the supermarket, armed with knowledge, and amused by the absurdity of some food labels. Ready to make choices that would delight a nutritionist, grab your reusable bags, and let's embark on this journey to detox your diet and elevate your eating game. It's time to transform your shopping trips into a triumphant march toward health and wellness!

Decoding the Ingredients

1. **Refined Sugars:**
   - **Sugar**
   - **Corn syrup**
   - **High-fructose corn syrup (HFCS)**
   - **Dextrose**
   - **Fructose**
   - **Sorbitol**

2. **Trans Fats:**
   - **Partially hydrogenated soybean oil**
   - **Mono and diglycerides**

3. **Saturated Fats:**

- Palm oil
- Whey protein concentrate

4. **Refined Carbohydrates:**
   - Enriched flour (wheat flour, niacin, reduced iron, thiamine mononitrate, riboflavin, folic acid)

5. **High Sodium:**
   - Sodium chloride
   - Monosodium glutamate (MSG)
   - Disodium inosinate
   - Disodium guanylate

6. **Artificial Additives and Preservatives:**
   - Sodium benzoate (preservative)
   - Artificial flavor
   - Color added (includes Yellow 5, Red 40)
   - Calcium propionate (preservative)
   - Butylated hydroxyanisole (BHA)
   - Butylated hydroxytoluene (BHT)

7. **High-Fructose Corn Syrup (HFCS):**
   - High-fructose corn syrup (HFCS)
   - Corn syrup

Explanation

- **Refined Sugars**: These are hidden under multiple names like sugar, corn syrup, high-fructose corn syrup, dextrose, fructose, and sorbitol, making it seem like the product contains less sugar than it actually does.

- **Trans Fats**: Partially hydrogenated oils and mono and diglycerides are often used to enhance texture and shelf life, but they contain harmful trans fats.

- **Saturated Fats**: Palm oil and whey protein concentrate

contribute to the saturated fat content, which can raise cholesterol levels.

- **Refined Carbohydrates**: Enriched flour is a refined carbohydrate that lacks the fiber and nutrients found in whole grains.

- **High Sodium**: Sodium chloride (table salt), MSG, disodium inosinate, and disodium guanylate are common additives that can contribute to high sodium intake.

- **Artificial Additives and Preservatives**: Sodium benzoate, artificial flavors, synthetic colors like Yellow 5 and Red 40, calcium propionate, BHA, and BHT are added to enhance flavor, color, and shelf life but may pose health risks.

- **High-Fructose Corn Syrup (HFCS)**: Both HFCS and corn syrup are used to sweeten the product, contributing to various health issues.

Recommended Brands:

Brands Committed to Health

Annie's Homegrown

- Where mac and cheese meet wholesome goodness, Annie ditches the artificial stuff for real ingredients that make your taste buds sing and your body rejoice.

Nature's Path

- A cereal brand that says no to GMOs and yes to organic, whole grains. It's like a crunchy hug for your morning routine.

Applegate

- Meat you can trust! Applegate serves up deli meats, sausages, and bacon without antibiotics or artificial ingredients. Because who needs mystery meat?

Bob's Red Mill

- Grain gurus! Bob's Red Mill offers everything from flour to oats, all-natural and minimally processed. Baking has never been so pure.

Eden Foods

- Beans, grains, and more! Eden Foods packs its products with organic goodness, avoiding harmful additives and embracing purity.

Amy's Kitchen

- Frozen food that feels like a home-cooked meal. Amy's crafts meals free from GMOs, artificial colors, and preservatives, making convenience nutritious.

KIND Snacks

- Bars that are kind to your body and the planet. KIND uses whole nuts, fruits, and grains, ensuring every bite is as wholesome as it is delicious.

Stonyfield Organic

- Yogurt that's good for you and the environment. Stonyfield's organic products avoid pesticides, GMOs, and artificial hormones, bringing you dairy delight.

Cascadian Farm

- Organic farming at its best! Cascadian Farm delivers cereals, granola bars, and frozen fruits and veggies, all grown with love and care for the planet.

Siggi's

- Yogurt that's not too sweet. Siggi keeps it simple with real fruit and minimal sugar, offering a creamy treat that's as nutritious as it is tasty.

Certification Labels

1. **USDA Organic**
   - The gold standard of organic certification. Products that bear this label must contain a minimum of 95% organic ingredients and must not include synthetic fertilizers, pesticides, or genetically modified organisms (GMOs). It's like a badge of honor for your food.

2. **Non-GMO Project Verified**
   - The butterfly seal of approval! This label guarantees that a product has undergone testing and is free of genetically modified organisms. It's your assurance that nature remains untampered.

3. **Certified Gluten-Free**
   - For those navigating the tricky world of gluten-free diets, this label ensures a product contains less than 20 parts per million of gluten, making it safe for individuals with celiac disease or gluten sensitivity. It's a peace of mind in a symbol.

4. **Fair Trade Certified**
   - A label that stands for ethical trade practices, fair wages, and sustainable farming. When you see this certification, you know the product supports better working conditions and community development. It's fair in every bite.

5. **Certified Humane**
   - This label guarantees farmers treated the animals used in the product humanely, providing ample space, shelter, and gentle handling. It's a symbol of compassion in animal farming.

6. **Rainforest Alliance Certified**

- Products with this certification contribute to conserving biodiversity and ensuring sustainable livelihoods for farmers. It's a promise of environmental stewardship.

7. **MSC Certified (Marine Stewardship Council)**
   - For seafood lovers, this label ensures that fish and seafood products come from sustainable and well-managed fisheries. It's an ocean-friendly choice that helps protect marine ecosystems.

8. **B Corp Certification**
   - More than just a food label, companies receive this certification for meeting high standards of social and environmental performance, accountability, and transparency. It's a mark of business for good.

9. **Kosher Certification**
   - This label signifies a product complies with Jewish dietary laws. Look for symbols like OU, Kof-K, or Star-K to ensure your food meets kosher standards.

10. **Halal Certification**
    - Products bearing this label comply with Islamic dietary laws, ensuring that the food is permissible (halal) for consumption. It's an assurance of faith-based dietary integrity.

Healthy Alternatives

1. **Maple Syrup** (Replaces: Refined Sugar)
   - Sweet, sticky, and natural! Maple syrup is nature's candy, perfect for drizzling on pancakes or adding to recipes without the

empty calories of refined sugar.

2. **Olive Oil** (Replaces: Partially Hydrogenated Oils/ Trans Fats)
   - Liquid gold from the Mediterranean! Use olive oil instead of those sneaky trans fats. It's heart-healthy and delicious for cooking, baking, or dressing salads.

3. **Avocado** (Replaces: Saturated Fats)
   - Creamy and dreamy! Avocado is the perfect swap for butter or cream. Spread it on toast, blend it into smoothies, or use it in baking for a healthy fat boost.

4. **Whole Wheat Flour** (Replaces: Refined Flour)
   - Grainy goodness! Whole wheat flour adds fiber and nutrients to your baking, making it a powerhouse substitute for refined, nutrient-stripped flour.

5. **Herbs and Spices** (Replaces: High Sodium/Salt)
   - Flavor explosion! Basil, oregano, cumin, and paprika bring zesty life to your dishes without the hypertension-inducing salt. Shake things up with these natural flavors!

6. **Natural Preservatives (Lemon Juice, Vinegar, Salt)** (Replaces: Artificial Additives and Preservatives)
   - Tangy and tart! Lemon juice and vinegar naturally preserve and flavor your foods, kicking artificial preservatives to the curb. Freshness and zest in every bite!

7. **Stevia** (Replaces: High-Fructose Corn Syrup)
   - Sweet without the spike! Stevia is a natural sweetener that won't send your blood sugar on a rollercoaster. Perfect for your tea, coffee, and baked goods.

8. **Coconut Sugar** (Replaces: Refined Sugar)
   - Island vibes! Coconut sugar has a lower glycemic index than refined sugar, offering

a caramel-like sweetness that's gentler on your blood sugar levels.

9. **Greek Yogurt** (Replaces: Sour Cream/Mayo)
   - Creamy delight! Greek yogurt is a protein-packed, probiotic-rich substitute for sour cream or mayo, adding tangy goodness to your dips, dressings, and baked potatoes.

10. **Quinoa** (Replaces: White Rice)
   - Protein-packed powerhouse! Quinoa is a nutrient-dense alternative to white rice, bringing complete protein and fiber to your meals.

Helpful Websites

1. **Fooducate** (www.fooducate.com)
   - Your personal nutritionist! Fooducate helps you decode food labels, giving each product a health grade. Scan barcodes and discover what's really inside your food. No more mystery ingredients!

2. **Environmental Working Group (EWG)** (www.ewg.org)
   - The watchdog of wellness! EWG's Food Scores rate over 80,000 products based on nutrition, ingredient concerns, and processing. It's like having a detective in your pocket.

3. **Eat This, Not That!** (www.eatthis.com)
   - The swap sensation! This website offers practical food swaps and advice for healthier eating. It's perfect for navigating grocery stores and restaurant menus with ease.

4. **Harvard T.H. Chan School of Public Health** (www.hsph.harvard.edu/nutritionsource)

- The brainy bunch! Harvard's Nutrition Source provides evidence-based advice on diet and nutrition. Stay informed with the latest research and tips.

Shopping Apps

1. **Shopwell**
   - Personalized perfection! Shopwell customizes your shopping experience based on your dietary needs. Scan items and get instant feedback on how they fit your nutritional goals.

2. **Yuka**
   - The healthy scanner! Yuka rates food and personal care products, highlighting their impact on your health. Scan a product, see the score, and make informed choices.

3. **HealthyOut**
   - Eating out, healthy HealthyOut helps you find restaurant meals that meet your dietary preferences. Whether it's gluten-free, low-carb, or vegan, this app has your back.

4. **Cronometer**
   - The ultimate tracker! Cronometer not only tracks your food intake but also gives detailed nutritional breakdowns. Monitor your macros, vitamins, and minerals with precision.

5. **MyFitnessPal**
   - The fitness friend! MyFitnessPal is a comprehensive app for tracking your diet and exercise. Log your meals, scan barcodes, and stay on top of your health goals.

Conclusion

With these online resources and apps, making healthy choices is just a click away. Equip yourself with the digital tools to navigate the grocery aisles, restaurants, and your own kitchen with confidence and ease. Embrace the tech-savvy way to a healthier you!

ABOUT THE AUTHOR

Kutu Maurus is a distinguished figure in human nutrition, holding a master's degree in human nutrition from the University of Bridgeport's rigorous nutrition institute in Connecticut, USA. As a certified nutritionist and personal trainer, Kutu brings a wealth of knowledge and expertise to the table, advocating for a holistic approach to health and wellness.

Kutu is a passionate advocate of holistic remedies and functional medicine, emphasizing the importance of treating the body as an integrated whole rather than merely addressing isolated symptoms. This belief extends to his fitness practice, where he promotes the benefits of calisthenics and lightweight training, promoting physical fitness that is both sustainable and accessible. As an amateur natural bodybuilder, Kutu exemplifies the power of nutrition and natural training methods in achieving peak physical condition without relying on performance-enhancing substances.

Besides his physical health expertise, Kutu is a fervent believer in the power of meditation and the mind's ability to aid in healing and maintaining health. His holistic approach encourages the integration of mental well-being with physical health, fostering a comprehensive path to wellness.

Kutu Maurus, an experienced educator, dedicates himself to sharing his knowledge and empowering others to take charge of their health through informed choices and mindful practices. This work, the "7 Deadly Ingredients" is a part of that mission. He has made significant contributions by working with private clients to help them achieve their health goals and by writing extensively on topics of health and wellness.

His teachings inspire individuals to embrace a balanced lifestyle that harmonizes body, mind, and spirit.

Kutu Maurus continues to make significant contributions to the field of nutrition and wellness, guiding countless individuals on their journey to optimal health and vibrant living.

My Departing Letter

Dear Beloved Readers,

As this journey ends, I am grateful for <u>ALL</u> of you and wish all the best on your path. I am truly humbled knowing you took the time to learn about how good your life can be - basking in a glow as warm and radiant, welcoming as light on a brand-new morning.

So far, we have explored the complex world of harmful ingredients to steer clear of and revealed all there is to learn (within the limits of this book) about nourishing your body without resorting to tasteless and bland foods.

We've explored the art of decisions, indulged in knowledge, and earned wisdom to master food geography. Your commitment to transformation and desire for a fulfilling life filled with continuous growth, rather than just focusing on facts and figures, is what truly illuminates the path forward.

I wanted to wish you the best on your journey forward. May you find glorious victories on your road to good health. Acknowledge and enjoy each positive step, knowing that every decision you make will get you one foot nearer to the glowing health and vitality that is your birthright.

Living healthily is one of humankind's most beautiful adventures. I pray you experience delight in eating, tasting the incredible immersion of natural flavors, and unlocking fresh paths to take care of yourself. May your kitchen be a place of joy and love in which you spend hours bent over the meals for yourself for those who are important too.

The essence of a fulfilling life is essential. May you start each day rejuvenated and full of eagerness, eager to embrace all the possibilities - whether ordinary or thrilling - and the everyday hurdles that exist in this world. There is great beauty and abundance within you, and your well-being should be so remarkable that it conveys a clear message of mindful decisions that others cannot overlook.

Just remember, you are not walking alone on this path. Indeed, you have a group of people with similar aspirations and a community who are just as passionate about health. Leverage them for support, get advice, and share what you are experiencing while motivating each other to keep going.

Finally, my beloved friends, I desire good health for you and a long life. May the days be so bright, your heart be light, and you soar in high spirits. You could turn your world around, one conscious choice at a time... Accept it with a full heart.

With the deepest gratitude, love, and warmest wishes,

Kutu

Please take the time to rate this book and comment. Please rate this book and leave a comment, as it will help more people find this information.

WORKS CITED

French, M. A., Sundram, K., & Clandinin, M. T. (2002). Cholesterolaemic effect of palmitic acid in relation to other. *Asia Pacific J Clin Nut, 11* (Suppl), S401–S407. Retrieved July 8, 2024, from https://apjcn.qdu.edu.cn/11_9_8.pdf

American Heart Association. ((2017). *The New American Heart Association Cookbook, 9th Edition: Revised and Updated with More Than 100 All-New Recipes.*. New York, NY.: Harmony.

American Heart Association. (2021, November 21). *Saturated Fats*. Retrieved July 8, 2024, from 100 Years American Heart Association: https://www.heart.org/en/healthy-living/healthy-eating/eat-smart/fats/saturated-fats#:~:text=The%20American%20Heart%20Association%20recommends, of %20saturated% 20fat% 20per% 20day.

American Heart Association. (2023, October 24). *Healthy Cooking Oils*. Retrieved July 8, 2024, from 100 Years American Heart Association: https://www.heart.org/en/healthy-living/healthy-eating/eat-smart/fats/healthy-cooking-oils

Blythman, J. (2015). *Swallow This: Serving Up the Food Industry's Darkest Secrets.*. London, England: Fourth Estate.

Campaign for Safe Cosmetics. (2024, July 4). *Laws and Regulations*. Retrieved from Campaign for Safe Cosmetics: https://www.safecosmetics.org/resources/regulations/

Can junk food alter your DNA? (2022, June 28). Retrieved from X Code Life: https://www.xcode.life/dna-and-nutrition/can-junk-food-alter-your-dna/

D'Elia, H., Rossi, G., Ippolito, A., Cappuccio, R., & Strazzullo, F. (2012). Salt intake and gastric cancer risk: A systematic review and meta-analysis. *Journal of Clinical Gastroenterology, 46*(1), 6-14. doi: https://doi.org/10.1097/MCG.0b013e318225dffb

Detrano, J. (2024, July 6). *Sugar Addiction: More Serious Than You*

Think. Retrieved from Rutgers University-The Center of Alcohol & Substance Use Studies: https://alcoholstudies.rutgers.edu/sugar-addiction-more-serious-than-you-think/

Erasmus, U. (1993). *Fats That Heal, Fats That Kill: The Complete Guide to Fats, Oils, Cholesterol, and Human Health..* Burnaby, BC.: Alive Books.

Fuhrman, J. (2018). The Hidden Dangers of Fast and Processed Food. *American Journal of Lifestyle Medicine*, Sep-Oct; 12(5): 375–381.

Hari, V. (2016). *The Food Babe Way.* New York: Little, Brown and Company.

Hyman, M. (2014). *The Blood Sugar Solution: The UltraHealthy Program for Losing Weight, Preventing Disease, and Feeling Great Now!.* New York: Little, Brown and Company.

Lustig, R. H. (2012). *Fat Chance: Beating the Odds Against Sugar, Processed Food, Obesity, and Diseas.* New York: Panguin Random House.

Mercola, J., & Pearsall, K. D. (2006). *Sweet Deception: Why Splenda, NutraSweet, and the FDA May Be Hazardous to Your Health.* Nashville, TN.: Thomas Nelson.

Mizel, J. (2023). *Mizel, J. (2013). The Fatty Liver Solution: TheEssential Guide to a Healthy Liver. CreateSpace Independent Publishing Platform.* Charleston, SC: CreateSpace Independent Publisher.

Moss, M. (2013). *Salt Sugar Fat: How the Food Giants Hooked Us.* New York: Random House.

Nestle, M. (2002). *Food Politics: How the Food Industry Influences Nutrition and Health.* Berkeley: University of California Press.

O'Brien, R., & Kranz,. R. (2009). *The Unhealthy Truth: One Mother's Shocking Investigation into the Dangers of America's Food Supply–and What Every Family Can Do to Protect Itself.* New York, NY.: Broadway Books.

Pollan, M. (2008). *In Defense of Food: An Eater's Manifesto. .* New York, NY.: Penguin Press.

Salvador, M. C., Aranda, A. P., & Fregapane, G. (2001). The influence of heating on the stability of extra virgin olive oil and the evolution of its antioxidant content. *Journal of Agricultural and Food Chemistry*, 49(12), 5705-5711. doi:10.1021/jf010792x

Schab, D. W., & Trinh, N.-H. (2004). Food additives and hyperactive behavior in children. *Journal of Developmental & Behavioral Pediatrics, 25*(6), 423-434.

Statham, B. (2007). *hat's in Your Food?: The Truth About Food Additives from Aspartame to Xanthan Gum.* Sydney, Australia: Running Press.

Taubes, G. (2016). *The Case Against Sugar.* New York: Alfred A. Knopf.

Teicholz, N. (2014). *The Big Fat Surprise: Why Butter, Meat and Cheese Belong in a Healthy Diet..* New York, NY.: Simon & Schuster.

Willett, W. C. (2017). *Eat, Drink, and Be Healthy: The Harvard Medical School Guide to Healthy Eating.* New York: Free Press; Reprint edition.

www.ingramcontent.com/pod-product-compliance
Lightning Source LLC
Chambersburg PA
CBHW050129280326
41933CB00010B/1310